LIVING

with

DEMENTIA

*A practical guide for families
and personal carers*

EDITED BY

ESTHER CHANG AND AMANDA JOHNSON

LIVING

with

DEMENTIA

*A practical guide for families
and personal carers*

ACER PRESS

First published 2013
by ACER Press, an imprint of
Australian Council *for* Educational Research Ltd
19 Prospect Hill Road, Camberwell, Victoria, 3124, Australia

www.acerpress.com.au
sales@acer.edu.au

Edited by Holly Proctor
Cover design, text design and typesetting by ACER Creative Services
Printed in Australia by McPherson's Printing Group

National Library of Australia Cataloguing-in-Publication entry:

Title: Living with dementia: a practical guide for families and
                              personal carers / edited by Esther Chang and Amanda Johnson.

ISBN: 9781742860442 (paperback)

Subjects: Dementia--Patients--Home care--Handbooks, manuals, etc.
                              Caregivers--Handbooks, manuals, etc.

Other Authors/Contributors: Chang, Esther, editor.
                              Johnson, Amanda, 1960- editor.

Dewey Number: 616.83

Disclaimer
This publication has been carefully reviewed and checked to ensure that the content is
as accurate and current as possible at the time of publication. We would recommend,
however, that the reader verifies any procedures, treatments, drug dosages or legal content
described in this book. Neither the editors, the contributors, nor the publisher assume
any liability for injury and/or damage to persons or property arising from any error in or
omission from this publication.

PEFC™
PEFC/21-31-16

The pages of this book are printed on paper derived
from forests promoting sustainable management.

FOREWORD

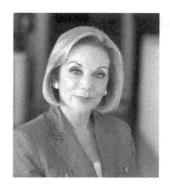

This book is a wonderful resource for carers of people with dementia; both family carers and paid carers. It provides many useful insights into the care and support of people with dementia.

We all know that dementia attacks the brain and impacts on a person's cognitive ability. The problem is, of course, that the symptoms vary greatly depending on an individual's age, characteristics and the parts of the brain most affected. For this reason, it is now well established that dementia care has to be person-centred and relate to the individual's personal needs as well as those of the family carer. It is so essential to understand the person's story and interests and how they have come to be the person they are. Good communication has to be centre stage and I am pleased that it has a chapter of its own in this publication.

The complexity and range of issues that need to be addressed are well illustrated by the range of topics in this book. These include the medical management of dementia, which is complex because of the many physical comorbidities that are associated with dementia including falls, delirium, weight loss, sleep disturbance and visual dysfunction.

Nevertheless, it is the lack of the acknowledgement of the role of the family carer that greatly concerns me. It is those closest to the person with dementia who are often best positioned to provide the insights necessary for diagnosis and the ongoing management of dementia.

It is important to keep in mind that about 60 per cent of people with dementia currently live in the community and there are more than one million Australians who provide support and care for a person with dementia. Their role can range from doing a little shopping or driving to 24-hour care.

I understand only too well the full-time responsibility, the juggling of priorities and the heartache that comes with caring for someone with dementia, having cared for my father when he was diagnosed with vascular dementia.

Perhaps the most difficult part of caring for someone with dementia is that the dementia itself is so unpredictable in the way that it affects individuals, the way it changes behaviours, emotions and the capacity of the individual to undertake tasks. Information and education are necessary prerequisites in preparing the family carer for what is to come in looking after someone with dementia but even so, the family carer can't anticipate the full import of assuming the roles and responsibilities that once were undertaken by the person with dementia.

The stress of caring for someone with dementia is often compounded by the stigma and social isolation that results from a diagnosis of dementia. As President of Alzheimer's Australia, I have had the opportunity of listening to carers' stories and have been told many times that the first outcome of the diagnosis has been a loss of contact with family and friends. It seems that social avoidance is the way that many people cope with dementia in our society rather than confronting how they might better understand and communicate with people with dementia and those who care for them.

The well-documented consequence is that the caring role inevitability takes its toll on the carer. Jane Thompson, who is a carer, has contributed to this book and captures the negative impact that caring for a person with dementia has on the carer's health and wellbeing. She emphasises the importance of respite.

I share the view that access to flexible respite services that provide good support for people with dementia and their carers is a high priority. Alzheimer's Australia is advocating that respite services should provide not only an important break for the carer but give the person with dementia the opportunity for social engagement and participation in meaningful activities.

This devastating condition has been negatively impacting on people's lives for too long. Although there is still much to be done, we should be proud that at the national level Australia is recognised as a world leader in tackling dementia. Bipartisan support has been an important part of our achievements and ongoing progress.

Consumers acknowledge the importance of workforce issues and the support and care that nurses and careworkers provide, often in difficult circumstances. Wages and conditions are often poor, as is access to training, and we know that there will be a desperate shortage of nurses and careworkers in aged care in the coming decades.

These challenges will compound the difficulty of improving the good quality care that those reading this book will be seeking to achieve.

For those seeking help, call the National Dementia Helpline on 1800 100 500 or visit the Alzheimer's Australia website at <www.fightdementia.org.au>.

Ita Buttrose AO, OBE
National President, Alzheimer's Australia

DEDICATION

*We wish to dedicate this book to all the carers
and families, in the hope it makes a difference to the lives
of people living with dementia.*

CONTENTS

PREFACE

From our research over the past decade, we have found that an information gap exists between paid and unpaid carers. It was, therefore, our desire to produce a book that is practical and helpful for both paid and unpaid carers. In the context of this book, a paid carer refers to a person who is employed by an organisation to deliver care in the community or in residential aged care facilities. An unpaid carer constitutes a family member or a person who has a caring relationship with the person with dementia and does not receive payment.

This book has been developed to provide reality-based and practical information for carers and families on key issues associated with caring for the person with dementia. It is divided into two parts: Part 1 discusses practical ways on how to care for the person with dementia and Part 2 offers guidance on how to communicate, examines how to care for the dying person and encourages and supports the carer from the perspective of a carer. Through reading this book, you will hopefully acquire insights into the complexities, challenges and concerns of living with dementia, as well as the opportunities. You will find viewpoints that are challenging, and sometimes confronting, but at the same time helpful and thought-provoking. We hope this reflection will create a shared understanding of the journey between you – the carer – and the person living with dementia. Importantly, understanding the whole person's response to their illness in the context of their own life history is pivotal to the provision of quality care. Enhanced understanding of dementia enables all involved to move beyond the negative perceptions frequently held about dementia to having hope that the person has a meaningful life within the limitations of the disease.

ACKNOWLEDGEMENTS

We extend our sincere appreciation to the contributors who share our interest and concern with the issues and challenges in caring for a person with dementia and we thank them for their work. This book would not have been possible without their commitment.

We would like to acknowledge Debbie Taylor Robson, at the University of Western Sydney, for her assistance in the initial stages of the manuscript. With thanks also to the reviewers, in particular, Tiffany Northall.

We wish to thank Debbie Lee, Managing Editor and Publisher, Holly Proctor, Project Editor, and the rest of the team at the Australian Council for Educational Research.

Finally, we would also like to thank our husbands, Ron and Robert, and our families for their support.

ABOUT THE EDITORS

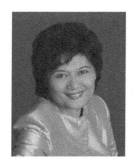

Professor Esther Chang is Director of the Higher Degree Research Program and Academic Course Advisor for the Honours Program in the School of Nursing and Midwifery, University of Western Sydney. Working in academia at various tertiary institutions since 1986, she has been a Head of School, Dean of the Faculty of Health and Acting Pro-Vice Chancellor Academic at the University of Western Sydney, Hawkesbury. Esther is committed to aged, dementia and palliative care and has received many large grants investigating nursing and health needs in older people and has developed models of care for acutely ill older patients and clients with end stage dementia. Esther's international links have also generated collaborative research into aged care across several countries. Pivotal to her academic and professional nursing knowledge is her personal experience caring for her mother who suffered from dementia and passed away in 2012.

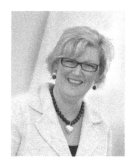

Dr Amanda Johnson is a Senior Lecturer (Aged Care) and Director of Academic Programs – Undergraduate at the School of Nursing and Midwifery, University of Western Sydney. Working in the tertiary sector since 1992, she has been an active leader in the development of undergraduate curriculum in the areas of aged care, chronic illness and palliation. In 2011, she completed her PhD thesis on undergraduate palliative care education and was the recipient of a Vice-Chancellor's Leadership Excellence Award for the Inherent Requirements of Nurse Education project. In 2010, she was Highly Commended in the Vice-Chancellor's Teaching Excellence Award for her curriculum development and teaching in the areas of chronic illness and palliation. Amanda strives to ensure that graduates are appropriately skilled and knowledgeable to provide quality care to older people and meet the challenges and complexities this poses through the leadership she provides in her teaching and research activities.

CONTRIBUTORS

Kaniez Baig, MB:BS, FRACGP, Clinical Safety Physician, bioCSL, Parkville, Vic.

Suzanne Brownhill, BSW, MPH, PhD, Research Fellow, School of Nursing and Midwifery, University of Western Sydney, NSW.

Esther Chang, RN, CM, DNE, BAppSci(Advanced Nursing), MEdAdmin, PhD, FCN, Professor of Nursing, Director of Higher Degree Research and Undergraduate Honours Programs, School of Nursing and Midwifery, University of Western Sydney, NSW.

Katherine L Cooper, RN, BN, MN, Lecturer in Nursing, Avondale College of Higher Education, NSW.

Lenore de la Perrelle, BA (SW), M.(Pol. Admin), Senior Manager, Dementia Learning and Development Unit, ACH Group, SA.

Michel Edenborough, PhD, BA, BSSc(Hons), Dip Mgmt, Cert IV Frontline Mgmt, Senior Research Officer, School of Nursing and Midwifery, University of Western Sydney, NSW.

Kathleen Dixon, RN, BA, MHA, PhD, Senior Lecturer, Director of Academic Workforce, School of Nursing and Midwifery, University of Western Sydney, NSW.

Rebecca Forbes, BIntStud, BA(Hons), Project Officer, The Dementia Centre, HammondCare, NSW.

Deborah Hatcher, RN, DipTeach(Phys.Ed), BHSc(N), MHPEd, PhD, Senior Lecturer, Director of Academic Workforce, School of Nursing and Midwifery, University of Western Sydney, NSW.

Anne Heard, BEd, GradDip (Group Work), Project Officer, Dementia Learning and Development Unit, ACH Group, SA.

Robyn Helm, RN, Diploma Business, Community Systems Manager, Baptist Community Services – NSW and ACT.

Kathryn G Goozee, NP, MCN, GDM, GCG, RN, Dementia Consultancy and Research Manager, Anglican Retirement Village, NSW and Adjunct Senior Lecturer, Edith Cowan University, WA.

Amanda Johnson, RN, DipT(Ng), MstHScEd, PhD, Senior Lecturer (Aged Care), Director of Academic Programs – Undergraduate, School of Nursing and Midwifery, University of Western Sydney, NSW.

Robert K Johnson, RN, MACM (UWS), BHA (UNSW), Cert Oncology, General Manager, Domain Principal Group, NSW.

Sara Karacsony, BA, RN, GradCert(Specialty Nursing), Clinical Nurse Specialist 2 Community Palliative Care, South Western Sydney Local Health District, NSW.

Danielle McIntosh, BAppSc(OT), MHlthServMgt, GradCert(Dementia Studies), Senior Dementia Consultant, The Dementia Centre, HammondCare, NSW.

Michelle McKinney, Cert IV Leisure and Lifestyle, Dip Mgmt, Lifestyle Consultant, Baptist Community Services – NSW and ACT.

Daniel Nicholls, RN, PhD, Associate Professor, Clinical Chair in Mental Health Nursing, ACT Health and Faculty of Health – Disciplines of Nursing & Midwifery, University of Canberra, ACT.

Shona P Nicholls, RN, RPN, CAdv Psych, BHSc, Clinical Nurse Consultant, Anglican Retirement Village, NSW.

Linda Ora, RN, MPallC, MACN, Clinical Nurse Consultant, Palliative Care, Primary Care and Community Health, Nepean Blue Mountains Local Health District, NSW.

Shyama G K Ratnayake, RN, MSc(Applied science), Research Officer, School of Nursing and Midwifery, University of Western Sydney, NSW.

Drene Somasundram, BA(Theology), MA(Education), DProf Doctorate in Professional Studies, Lecturer and Chaplain, Avondale College of Higher Education, NSW.

Jane Thompson, BSc(Hons), MSc, PhD, Visiting Fellow, Australian National University Medical School, ACT.

Karen Watson, BN(Hons), BHlthSc(Naturopathy), Registered Nurse, Carrington Centennial Care, NSW.

JOURNEYS WITH DEMENTIA

Esther Chang
University of Western Sydney

Amanda Johnson
University of Western Sydney

Chapter outcomes

When you have completed this chapter you will be able to:

- ▸ gain a shared understanding of what it means to care for a person living with dementia, which will assist you in becoming empowered and informed
- ▸ better understand the dementia journey you will co-share with the person living with dementia
- ▸ acquire insights into the complexities and challenges of living with dementia.

Keywords

journeys, dementia, challenges, support, carers

Introduction

This chapter attempts to increase the awareness of the many challenges a person living with and dying with dementia presents to family and professional carers. It is important to understand the whole person's response to their illness in the context of their own life history. Better understanding of dementia enables all involved to move beyond the negative perceptions held of dementia to having hope in a person developing a meaningful life within the limitations of the disease.

The person with dementia's journey is likened to travelling from a state of wellness and independence to one resulting in complete dependence and loss of self. This journey can take many roads and forms, which means that living with dementia is individual to each person. By its very nature, the journey that dementia takes people on means they need to adapt and adjust to the changes in how their body responds physically, mentally, spiritually and emotionally. People with dementia who embrace these changes are more likely to have a life that has some meaning, within a cognitive, social and functionally declining context.

The person with dementia's self is redefined by the nature of the disease and part of the journey is about how best their social network of family and carers can support the individual. The involvement of family, friends and professional carers in the care of people living with dementia is invaluable, regardless of where the care is provided. Sharing care helps to maintain the best possible quality of life of the person with dementia. Living with and caring for a person who has dementia and who will ultimately die presents both a crisis and a challenge to family and friends, who will be required to adjust and adapt their roles and functions in light of changes the person with dementia experiences (Johnson, 2012). Embracing these changes forges a reshaping of the lives of all those connected with the person who has dementia.

Dementia is on the increase and becoming a burdensome health issue (Deloitte Access Economics, 2011). It is a highly debilitating, progressive and life-limiting disease, with a trajectory ranging from approximately two to 20 years (Palliative Care Dementia Interface, 2011). While a person with dementia may not die of the disease they will unquestionably die with it. The disease is acknowledged as being terminal and is likened to a cancer diagnosis. However, this recognition has been slow and it is only now that a body of evidence is emerging (Chang & Johnson, 2012; Chang et al., 2013; Hancock et al., 2006). Worldwide, 35.6 million people have some form of dementia with 4.6 million new cases diagnosed each year (Alzheimer's Disease International,

2010). In Australia, there are currently 266 574 people affected by dementia, predicted to reach 942 624 people by the year 2050 (Deloitte Access Economics, 2011).

In presenting this chapter, the term 'journeys' is used to illustrate the three phases of dementia: starting the journey; being on the journey; and the journey's ending. The idea of journeying in three phases is informed by the work of Small, Froggatt and Downs (2008) and is a concept commonly used in caring for dying people. The phases of the journey are not separate or unconnected; there are numerous overlaps, as the journey takes many paths and is never in a straight line.

Journeys for the person with dementia

What is dementia?

Dementia is a disease of the brain that involves the brain cells being injured. There are many diseases that can cause dementia and other external factors that may contribute to a person developing dementia (McKeel et al., 2007). The most common types of dementia are Alzheimer's disease (50% of cases) and vascular dementia (20% of cases) (Access Economics, 2010). Alzheimer's disease occurs when brain cells are damaged. Gradually more and more brain cells fail to work properly and the result is a slow decline of mental powers (NHS Health Scotland, 2009). In vascular dementia, the blood supply to the brain is damaged or interrupted in some way. In multi-infarct dementia, tiny strokes (called infarcts) cut off the blood supply to small areas of the brain and the brain cells die (NHS Health Scotland, 2009). Losing brain cells means the person's brain does not work as well as it should. Gradually the person begins to lose the ability to do everyday activities. Often it affects memory first. The person may be confused about where they are, what day it is and who they are. Everyday tasks then become more difficult to undertake and their personality may change (NHS Health Scotland, 2009.) It is a sad fact that people with dementia will have a shortened life span because of their condition. As dementia progresses, the brain stops working properly. As the brain controls all bodily organs and systems, they too are affected and as these systems fail, a variety of medical complications occur and death is the inevitable outcome (Palliative Care Dementia Interface, 2011).

Stages of dementia

When people talk about dementia or you read about dementia they may refer to different stages of dementia. A 'stage' is simply a term used to conveniently describe a group of behaviours and medical issues that tend to occur together as dementia progresses. The terms that are used are mild, moderate, severe and end stage dementia. Advanced dementia is the term used to denote a combination of both severe and end stages of the disease. Regardless of the stage the person with dementia is in, pivotal to their care is a need for communication between the person with dementia, their family and carers.

Communication and dementia

Most people are filled with emotions when they discover that their family member or friend has dementia. Some are relieved to finally know the cause of the strange behaviour, while others are fearful of losing their loved one or feel helpless from not knowing how to communicate with them.

As the person with dementia declines, their capacity to be able to speak and understand what is being said diminishes. It is very important to be aware of this, particularly in the advanced stage of dementia where it is most difficult for the person's needs to be expressed and how best they can be supported while dying may not be addressed (Johnson et al., 2009). Furthermore, having other diseases and/or disabilities, such as poor eyesight, hearing impairment or heart failure, may also impede the person's ability to communicate. Maintaining and sustaining some sense of verbal and/or non-verbal connection with the person is equally important for the wellbeing of the family and carers as it is for the person regardless of the stage of the disease and the presence of other conditions or disabilities.

People with dementia experience a range of communication issues that may be unique to the individual. These issues may present as:

- being confused
- failing to recognise familiar objects
- being apathetic through displaying a lack of interest in everyday activities
- losing the ability to speak
- failing to know where they are, who they are and who you are
- expressing their feelings in ways they may not have previously, such as anger, frustration, anxiety and fear
- getting fixed on a particular way of saying things or repeating it over and over
- having issues with their memory, which means they cannot hold a conversation with another person or they can't recall your conversation from the day before.

These are just some of the examples you and the person with dementia may experience to a lesser or greater degree.

Knowing the person

Knowing who the person is assists paid carers to better understand the person with dementia's life history and their needs, which is more likely to lead to enhanced communication with the person and their family.

There are many ways in which communication between the person with dementia, their family and carers can be enabled. These strategies include but are not limited to: removing unwanted stimuli; getting into the right position; promoting equal participation; promoting the person to speak and engage in the conversation regardless of their limits; providing opportunities to talk; being sensitive to non-verbal clues; valuing and respecting contributions; and promoting joint decision-making and care planning (Adams & Gardiner, 2005). Family and carers frequently find that their role is about coaching the person to express their fears and concerns, to seek out the information they need to have a sense of control and to adjust to their changing life circumstances.

Establishing open communication between the person with dementia, their family and carers from the outset of the diagnosis is very important as this will assist when trying to determine their wishes for future care (Johnson et al., 2009). Over the course of the disease, the person may have an impaired capacity to make decisions. What constitutes the capacity to make decisions about health care is a contentious issue. The person is presumed to have the capacity to make their own decisions until this is proven otherwise. In the severe and end stages of the disease, however, another person will need to make all decisions on behalf of the person with dementia. Therefore, if the person's wishes are known in advance, and are discussed and planned for, this better supports all involved and enables the person to be active in the decisions related to their care. It also means the burden of making decisions becomes a shared responsibility with the person who has dementia, their family and carers.

Starting the journey

There is now evidence to indicate that people with dementia are conscious of the problems they are experiencing before the condition is diagnosed (Froggatt 1988; Moniz–Cook et al., 2006). Some experience memory loss, cognitive symptoms and functional impairments and describe a concern with 'losing their mind' or 'going mad' (Small et al., 2008, p. 27). One person with dementia described 'feeling as though a fog was covering his mind, making it hard to think clearly' (NHS Health Scotland, 2008, p. 14). A person's realisation that there is something wrong may sometimes lead them to the acceptance of practical strategies to manage their lives. However, the person in the early stages of dementia may start to withdraw from social interactions so that people will not notice the changes. A diagnosis formalises what they have been experiencing. The person with dementia also needs emotional and practical support. Talk to your doctor or another health or social work professional about this. Perhaps the person could see a counsellor to assist them to cope with the diagnosis.

Not everyone will get dementia in old age. Old age does not cause dementia but it is more common in older people; that is, people 65 years of age or older. However, we are also seeing younger onset dementia (YOD), which is dementia of any form that is diagnosed in people under the age of 65 years. Approximately 6.2% of the total population has younger onset dementia (Access Economics, 2010). If you are aware, however, of someone who is forgetful, confused or agitated, do not assume that they have dementia. Memory loss or confusion can sometimes be caused by infections, medications (such as sleeping pills), stress, anxiety and sometimes depression.

Selena's mother, Nancy, is in the early stages of vascular dementia and at times becomes disoriented. Selena sometimes feels sad and sometimes angry as she deals with the many symptoms of her mother's illness. However, she realises that when she expresses her frustration or reprimands her mother, this tends to result in childlike behaviour. Selena has therefore learnt to deal with her unpleasant feelings and has developed coping mechanisms that are also beneficial to her mother. Rather than speaking to her as though she were a child, Selena now tries to maintain a respectful adult-to-adult relationship.

Being on the journey

Being on the journey involves moving from the time dementia is diagnosed through the various stages until death. It may also mean requiring different care in a range of settings during the course of the disease such as home care, acute hospital care and residential aged care. The progress of the disease does not follow a set pattern or time period. This means that no one can give definite answers regarding what to expect. The problems and issues that arise from dementia occur from day to day and hour to hour. Each change requires adjustment. As dementia progresses, the person with dementia may become forgetful and will be likely to repeat things. They may understand that they have dementia or may realise something is wrong and often become anxious. The ability to talk is steadily lost, until only a few words are left or the person becomes mute and unable to speak at all. Instead of talking, people with dementia sometimes make strange sounds or even scream. If this happens, it usually means they are trying to communicate something such as they are uncomfortable (for example, they may be hot, cold or in pain). Family members and other carers who know them well can usually work out what is wrong and help them to settle.

> *Mr Lee is a 75-year-old Malaysian man, who was diagnosed with Alzheimer's dementia eight years ago. He has a wife and three adult children. He has just been admitted to a residential aged care facility (RACF) because of his behavioural problems. The general practitioner had become concerned about his wandering, his increasingly aggressive manner and the potential of falls. On visiting Mr Lee at the RACF, his wife and son became quite distressed because at first he failed to recognise them. Fortunately, a staff member who was nearby was able to explain that moving to a new environment can sometimes cause the person with dementia to become disoriented. This explanation helped Mrs Lee and her son to better accept the situation. They sat quietly with Mr Lee and gave him the opportunity to gradually adjust and reconnect.*

Ending the journey

People with dementia may choose to actively engage with their illness and the experiences it brings, while others may not. Family and carers may also become isolated from people. This often happens if the person with dementia behaves in an embarrassing way. The presence of dementia has major implications for the person; for their living and dying. The types of decisions made by carers and family members are influenced by their understanding of dementia as a terminal illness. For many carers, looking after someone with dementia brings changes in family relationships (Johnson, 2012; Small et al., 2008). As the illness goes on, the changes are greater and memory problems can worsen. The person's behaviour can also change and sometimes understanding or coping with this is hard. Despite good care, and regardless of where that care is given, the time will come when the person with dementia becomes so sick that they are likely to die. No one can tell you exactly when death will occur. In the final stages of dementia, signs such as swallowing problems, weight loss and increased immobility and muscle weakness together point to the fact that the general health of the person is getting worse. Eventually no amount of treatment, even if the person is in hospital, will prolong life (Chang et al., 2009; Palliative Care Dementia Interface, 2011). If the individual is in a residential care facility or hospital and the staff see that their medical condition is deteriorating, they are likely to contact the family members and other people close to the dying person to talk to them about what is happening. The family and significant others will usually be given the choice to stay with the dying person.

> *Soon after her diagnosis of Alzheimer's disease, Jenny sat down with her husband Anthony to discuss her Advance Care Plan. The plan included her wishes regarding end-of-life treatment, such as tube feeding and resuscitation, knowing that such decisions would likely be required at some stage in the future. Anthony realised he could not control the illness, nor could he prevent the deterioration of Jenny's condition, but having a plan in place gave them both considerable peace of mind. As heartbreaking as it was, it was also essential for Anthony to find a way of accepting the loss and letting Jenny go, a little bit each day. He made an effort not to deny his feelings of pain and sadness, but instead drew great strength from his network of friends and family who supported him while he continued to care for his wife. After Jenny died, Anthony took solace from the fact that he and Jenny had planned ahead and that her wishes had been respected.*

Conclusion

In this chapter, we have sought to present accounts of the journey of living and dying with dementia. This journey can take many roads and forms, with no one path determined. This means that how people live with dementia is individual to each person. For most people that are caring for someone with dementia, day-to-day living becomes the most important goal as they journey with the disease and try to make the person's life meaningful. Caring for someone with dementia can affect your social life, work life, financial situation and family relationships. The long journey has both positive and challenging experiences and it varies between individuals over time. Do not try to cope on your own. It will be a challenging journey because of the multitude of ways dementia impacts on the person's life and family. To be able to carry out your role as a carer you need to maintain your own physical, spiritual and emotional health. Being conscious about your diet and exercise and ensuring you get enough sleep will keep you strong and help you to maintain your resilience. Taking time off from caring duties and having time away from the person you care for is also important. This may involve seeking assistance and support from services for everyday caring needs.

References

Access Economics. (2010). *Caring places: Planning for aged care and dementia 2010–2050* (Vol. 2). Prepared for Alzheimer's Australia. Retrieved from http://www.fightdementia.org.au/common/files/NAT/20110225_Nat_AE_CaringPlacesV2.pdf

Adams, T. (2008). Communication between people with dementia, family members and nurses. In T. Adams (Ed.), *Dementia care nursing: Promoting well-being in people with dementia and their families* (pp. 144–161). Hampshire, UK: Palgrave Macmillan.

Adams, T., & Gardiner, P. (2005). Communication and interaction within dementia care triads: Developing a theory for relationship centred care. *Dementia: The international journal of social research and practice, 4*(2), 185–205.

Alzheimer's Disease International. (2010). *World Alzheimer report 2010: The global economic impact of dementia.* Retrieved from http://www.alz.co.uk/research/files/WorldAlzheimerReport2010.pdf

Chang, E., & Johnson, A. (2012). Challenges in advanced dementia. In E. Chang & A. Johnson (Eds.), *Contemporary and Innovative Practice in Palliative care* (pp. 151–164). Rijeka, Croatia: InTech Books.

Chang, E., Johnson, A., & Hancock, K. (2013). Advanced Dementia. In E. Chang & A. Johnson (Eds.), *Chronic illness and disability: Principles for nursing practice* (2nd ed.). Sydney: Elsevier.

Chang, E. M., Daly, J., Johnson, A., Harrison, K., Easterbrook, S., Bidewell, J., Stewart, H., Noel, M., & Hancock, K. (2009). Challenges for professional care of advanced dementia. *International Journal of Nursing Practice, 15*(1), 41–47.

Deloitte Access Economics. (2011). *Dementia across Australia: 2011–2050.* Prepared for Alzheimer's Australia. Retrieved from http://www.fightdementia.org.au/research-publications/access-economics-reports.aspx

Froggatt, A. (1988). Self-awareness in early dementia. In B. Gearing, M. Johnson & T. Heller (Eds.), *Mental health problems in old age: A reader* (pp. 131–136). Chichester, UK: John Wiley and Sons.

Hancock, K., Chang, E., Johnson, A., Harrison, K., Daly, J., Easterbrook, S., Noel, M., Davidson, P. (2006). Palliative care for people with advance dementia: The need for a collaborative evidence-based approach. *Alzheimer's Care Quarterly, 7*(1), 49–57.

Johnson, A. (2012). Families. In M. O'Connor, S. Aranchia & S. Lee (Eds.), *Palliative care: A guide to practice* (pp. 256–269). Ascot Vale, Vic.: Ausmed.

Johnson, A., Chang, E., Daly, J., Harrison, K., Noel, M., Hancock, K., Easterbrook, S. (2009). The communication challenges faced in adopting a palliative care approach in advance dementia. *International Journal of Nursing Practice, 15*(5), 467–474.

McKeel, D.W., Burns, J. M., Meuser, T. M., & Morris, J. C. (2007). *Dementia: An atlas of investigation and diagnosis.* Oxford, UK: Clinical Publishing.

Moniz-Cook, E., Manthorpe, J., Carr, I., Gibson, G., Vernooij-Dassen, M. (2006). Facing the future: A qualitative study of older people referred to memory clinic prior to assessment and diagnosis. *Dementia: The International Journal of Social Research and Practice, 4*(3), 442–449.

NHS Health Scotland. (2009). *Coping with dementia: A practical handbook for carers.* Edinburgh: NHS Health Scotland. Retrieved from http://www.healthscotland.com/uploads/documents/15905-CopingWithDementia2009.pdf

Palliative Care Dementia Interface: Enhancing Community Capacity Project. (2011). *Dementia: Information for families and friends of people with severe and end stage dementia* (3rd ed.). Sydney: University of Western Sydney.

Small, N., Froggatt, K., & Downs, M. (2008). *Living and dying with dementia.* Oxford: Oxford University Press.

Part 1

UNDERSTANDING HOW TO CARE: ACTIVITIES FOR DAILY LIVING

Chapter 1

SENSORY FUNCTIONS

Robyn Helm
Baptist Community Services – NSW and ACT

Michelle McKinney
Baptist Community Services – NSW and ACT

Chapter outcomes

When you have completed this chapter you will be able to:

- understand the changes that occur to the senses as people age
- include sensory stimulus in everyday practice for a person with dementia
- use sensory activities to enhance lifestyle experiences and increase social interactions for the carer and the person with dementia.

Keywords

sight, hearing, touch, smell, taste

Introduction

As people age their sensory functions gradually deteriorate. This can reduce a person's sense of wellbeing and build on the existing sense of isolation that often occurs for the person with dementia. It is well known that hearing and vision impairments are associated with a decline in physical and social functioning among the older person (Fischer et al., 2009), therefore, the loss of sensory functions is one of the most significant negative implications of ageing. Fulfilling experiences of enjoyment and wellbeing for a person with dementia may be limited through reduced vision and hearing, a lack of touch and smell and reduced perceptions of taste.

Hearing impairment causes difficulties in most situations in which interpersonal communication is needed. Reduced hearing and visual capacities are also found to be detrimental for both communication and orientation (Bergman & Rosenhall, 2001). Some of this can be alleviated by providing sensory stimulus. To stimulate the senses is to provide a stimulus to all or any one of the five senses. This can be done through recreational activities and therapies or through creative ways of engaging the person with dementia in the general activities of daily living.

Multisensory environments can be used to assist the stimulation of the senses. Collier et al. (2010) used gardening as an activity-based intervention to provide comparable multisensory stimulation through sight, hearing, touch, taste and smell. Activities such as gardening support those with dementia in coping with confusion and behaviour changes that are consequences of progressive, debilitating illness (Collier et al., 2010). Sensory activities have the ability to increase social engagement, lifestyle enjoyment and improve interactions between the carer and the person with dementia.

Sight

As ageing occurs it is very common for eyesight to change too. One study found that people who had trouble 'reading small print or recognising people across the street were more likely to have an age-related eye disease' (Knudson et al., 2005, p. 807). Visual changes usually start when a person reaches their forties. Many older people experience some decrease in their vision and may need to wear glasses. It is important to ensure the person with dementia has regular eye checks to determine their level of vision and to check for macular degeneration or the presence of cataracts. The carer may need to encourage the person with dementia to wear their glasses and to assist with keeping their glasses clean on a daily basis.

Impaired vision can lead to falls and a sense of disorientation as well as contributing to a sense of isolation for the person with dementia so it's important that it is addressed. Visual impairment can also be linked to individuals with dementia not attending social or religious activities, which are important markers for social isolation in the older community (West et al., 1997).

The environment is an important factor in maximising vision. Some simple guidelines to follow when looking at the environment for a person with dementia include ensuring the area is uncluttered, clean, well lit and inviting. This will help to reduce the person's potential of falling and their feelings of confusion. Lighting should be effective and evenly distributed throughout all rooms. Sensor lights can be purchased to ensure areas are lit at night if the person with dementia is inclined to get up or wander.

Signs that are easy to read can be placed on the doors of bathrooms in the home or aged care facilities. It is suggested that doors and walls are painted a different colour to ensure the door stands out and the person with dementia knows where to go. It is also recommended that there is a contrast in colour between furnishings and the floor to maximise any visual deficits the person with dementia might have. This is true for furniture and soft furnishings too. These simple steps will assist in promoting independence and dignity for the person with dementia.

Familiarity with the environment is important to the person with dementia and may reduce anxiety and wandering. If the person with dementia is in an unfamiliar space it is important to have recognisable items from their home that will promote positive memories.

Other ideas for visual stimulation include artwork, interesting light effects such as lava lamps and stained glass windows, brightly coloured clothing, fish tanks, digital photo frames and photograph albums. All of these items can be used to encourage discussion and trigger memories. In particular, digital photo frames and photograph albums provide an avenue for reminiscence, an activity enjoyed by older people and people with dementia. Large print books and magazines can also be used as discussion points to engage the person with dementia.

Whatever the method used, it is important to remember that the visual stimulation needs to be person-centred.

Hearing

There are several issues related to hearing loss in the person with dementia. As a first step, when communicating with the person with dementia, the carer needs to focus on the person. They need to speak clearly, listen and face the person as they speak. This will help the person to see that the carer is speaking to them.

Exposure to constant loud noise can compound the normal hearing loss that occurs with age. Hearing loss makes communication difficult particularly in group situations or where there is a lot of background noise. If the person with dementia is enjoying an activity, or is busy with a task, it is important to minimise all background distractions. Ringing telephones and noisy televisions can be distressing to the person with dementia, whereas soft background music, such as baroque music, may be effective in creating a calm environment. Research varies on this outcome but it might be worthwhile trying when considering person–centred musical activities.

Regular hearing checks and encouragement or physical assistance to wear their hearing aids will assist the person with dementia in communicating and gaining the most out of sensory experiences. Carers may need to assist in ensuring hearing aids are clean and the batteries are in good working order.

Carers can use various methods to stimulate the hearing of the person with dementia. Hearing stimulation has the potential to improve communication and interaction and provide enjoyment and fun for the person. An example of this is the use of music therapy.

Music has the power to trigger emotions and memories for people with dementia. One research study concluded that the presence of music, through enhancing a general level of activation, may prompt motor activity or memory recall (Cuddy & Duffin, 2005). For this reason, many aged care facilities employ a music therapist. Music therapy is a creative way of using music with the aim of optimising and maintaining health and wellbeing in an individual. Singing is also a popular and an enjoyable pastime for many carers and people with dementia. At times people with advanced dementia have been able to sing songs when their ability to speak seems to be lost. When using any form of music as an activity, the musical choices should be those of the person with dementia.

Taste

There is little change in taste as we age, although poor dental hygiene, some medications and existing physical and psychological symptoms can affect the enjoyment a person with dementia has in eating. This reduced enjoyment has the potential to reduce the nutritional status of the person and may result in weight loss and poor health outcomes. Causes of weight loss in older people can be classified as 'organic (e.g. neoplastic, nonneoplastic and age-related changes), psychological (e.g. depression, dementia, anxiety disorders) or nonmedical (e.g. socioeconomic conditions)' (Alibhai, Greenwood & Payette, 2005, p. 773). There are some simple things the carer can do to assist the person with dementia when wanting to heighten taste and improve nutritional outcomes. Good dental hygiene is one of the most important. Regular visits to the dentist, twice daily teeth cleaning and ensuring that dentures fit well will help the taste experience.

It is also important to remember that eating is more than just consuming food. For most of us it is a social experience as well. Make the meal experience more meaningful by providing an inviting environment for the person with dementia. Soft background music and an appealing table setting and tablecloth will make a difference to any meal. Finger foods may be more appealing than a large plate of food. When weight loss is an issue make sure there are opportunities for eating outside of the usual mealtimes to assist with building the number of kilojoules the person with dementia has each day. Fruit platters and ice cream trolleys (a reminder of past cinema experiences) may provide a fun happy hour in an aged care facility. To encourage the person with dementia to eat and enjoy the experience, ensure food does not look bland on the plate but is bright and colourful with a variety of food groups. This colour palette should apply to pureed food as well. Cooking demonstrations are a good activity in aged care facilities where the person with dementia gets to taste the end product. Hold a high tea with teapots, teacups and different snacks to taste or involve the person in the tasting of different herbs and vegetables in the garden. This can be a meaningful activity and is something that has the potential to enhance socialisation and relationship building. More detail concerning eating and swallowing can be found in Chapter 3.

A physiotherapist may help to increase the amount of exercise the person with dementia does, thereby stimulating appetite and increasing energy intake and muscle mass (Alibhai et al., 2005). Daily walks can also help and have the potential to increase the rapport between the carer and the person with dementia.

Touch

Anecdotally, we hear of people being starved of touch as they age. One study found that spending a few moments using touch with people who live with dementia, women in particular, opens up the possibility of discovering significant psychological capacities that may have previously remained untapped or hidden (Trotman & Brody, 2002). Therapeutically, touch between two individuals 'establishes and intensifies psychological connectedness' and enhances the communication of information and understanding (Trotman & Brody, 2002, p. 184). Women who may have been wives and mothers and who were pivotal to the running of a home and family may no longer have access to the warmth of touch. People in an aged care facility may only experience touch when a procedure is being done to them, for example, wound dressings or personal hygiene.

There has been some research to suggest that massage and touch interventions can be effective alternative treatments for people with dementia in helping to counteract anxiety, agitated behaviour, depression and possibly to slow down cognitive decline. Unfortunately, there is little documented evidence to back up these claims, in part because only limited research has been undertaken. One study (Holey & Cook, 2004) found that hand massage and music may have some short-term benefits in reducing agitated behaviour and that a gentle touch on the arm, followed by verbal encouragement, can increase the intake of kilojoules for a person with dementia. Hand massages can also promote 'social interaction and shared enjoyment' (Holey & Cook, 2004, p. 315). It is worthwhile trying these suggestions to see if the person with dementia receives some positive benefits.

Touch can be a very personal sense and carers need to be intuitive as to the amount of touch an individual enjoys. Remember, touch does not need to be restricted to skin-to-skin. There are many ways touch can be introduced into the lives of people with dementia but a person-centred approach should always be used.

One Baptist Community Services (NSW and ACT) aged care facility holds a weekly philosophy group that meets to discuss different topics such as feminism and religion. The purpose of the group is to encourage intellectual discussion and thoughts about local and world issues. At the end of the discussion participants have a choice of receiving a chocolate or a hug from the facilitator. Most often, the preferred choice is a hug over receiving a chocolate. This is indicative of how much many older people appreciate physical displays of care, understanding and support. Paid carers need to be aware of specific organisational policy in relation to their display of physical interaction and touch with residents.

Some suggestions for enhancing the sense of touch include creating sensory boxes that contain a variety of objects, for example, feathers, fabrics, sand and shells, that can be touched and then discussed. Massages, facials and hair brushing may also be soothing to someone who enjoys the experience. Developing a sensory garden with plants that impact on all the senses or taking a walk in a garden or park and touching leaves, tree trunks, grass and flowers may be relaxing. Tools or gardening implements might also be good to handle, discuss and bring back old memories. The feel of warm water can provoke fun and laughter and bring back memories of holidays and sunshine. There is also some evidence that pet therapy assists in alleviating depression and promoting laughter and wellbeing. If pets are not possible, baby dolls and robotic animals may be an avenue to explore.

Smell

The sense of smell gradually declines as a normal part of ageing. Many people are not even aware that they have a problem with their sense of smell because the changes occur gradually over several years. The person may not even notice that they are experiencing a loss of smell until there is an incident; for example, where they didn't detect food that had burnt or weren't aware of the presence of smoke. The loss of the sense of smell is more common than the loss of taste, and many older people mistakenly believe they have a problem with taste, when they are really experiencing a problem with their sense of smell. The loss of taste perception in sweet and salty foods can have health consequences for the older person (Schiffman, 1997). When smell is impaired, it is natural for people to change their eating habits. Some may eat too little and lose weight while others may eat too much and gain weight. The loss of the sense of smell may also cause people to complain about their food as tasteless or cause them to add extra salt to improve the taste. This is an area to be aware of when people with dementia are losing weight and not eating adequately. A collection of perfume cards can be very effective at bringing back memories of department store shopping or dressing up for special occasions. Cooking aromas, such as freshly baked bread, bacon and eggs, coffee and baked dinners, are popular and may be very familiar to the person with dementia. Men might enjoy smells that bring back memories of their garage or shed. Suggestions include car, machinery and tool smells. Many people also enjoy the smell of gardens and freshly cut grass, spring flowers, citrus fruits and mangoes.

Conclusion

This chapter serves as a guide to the senses and the impact they have on enhancing wellbeing, and a sense of enjoyment for the person with dementia. When looking at any method of sensory stimulus the focus needs to be on the individual preferences of the person with dementia ensuring that all approaches are person-centred.

References

Alibhai, S. M. H., Greenwood, C., & Payette, H. (2005). An approach to the management of unintentional weight loss in elderly people. *Canadian Medical Journal, 172*(6), 773–780.

Bergman, B., & Rosenhall, U. (2001). Vision and hearing in old age. *Scandinavian Audiology, 30*(4), 255–263.

Collier, L., McPherson, K., Ellis-Hill, C., Staal, J, & Bucks, R. (2010). Multisensory stimulation to improve functional performance in moderate to severe dementia – interim results. *American Journal of Alzheimer's Disease and Other Dementias, 25*(8), 698–703.

Cuddy, L. L., & Duffin, J. (2005). Music, memory and Alzheimer's disease: Is music recognition spared in dementia and how can it be assessed? *Medical Hypotheses, 64*(2), 229–235.

Fischer, M. E., Cruickshanks, K. J., Klein, B. E. K., Klein, R., Schubert, C. R., & Wiley, T. L. (2009). Multiple sensory impairment and quality of life. *Ophthalmic Epidemiology, 16*(6), 346–353.

Holey, E., & Cook, E. (2004). *Evidence-based therapeutic massage: A practical guide for therapists.* London: Elsevier Health.

Knudson M. D., Klein, B. E., Klein, R., Cruickshanks, K. J., & Lee, K. E. (2005). Age-related eye disease, quality of life and functional activity. *Archives of Ophthalmology, 123*(6), 807–814.

Schiffman, S. S. (1997). Taste and smell losses in normal ageing and disease. *Journal of the American Medical Association, 278*(16), 1357–1373.

Trotman, F. K., & Brody, C. M. (2002). *Psycho-therapy and counselling with older women: Cross-cultural, family and end-of-life issues.* New York: Springer Publishing Co.

West, S. K., Munoz, B., Rubin, G. S., Schein, O. D., Bandeen-Roche, K., Zeger, S., German, S., & Fried, L. P. (1997). Function and visual impairment in a population-based study of older adults. The SEE project: Salisbury Eye Evaluation. *Investigative Ophthalmology & Visual Science, 38*(1), 72–82.

Chapter 2

PERSONAL HYGIENE AND GROOMING

Robert K Johnson
Domain Principal Group

Chapter outcomes

When you have completed this chapter you will be able to:

▶ better assess and respond to the needs of the person with dementia for personal hygiene and grooming

▶ use strategies for the practical care of the person with dementia and maintenance of their independence

▶ better understand what can be expected as the disease progresses and its effect on the functioning of the person with dementia.

Keywords

bathing, dressing, hair care, oral care, nail care

Introduction

Personal hygiene and grooming fall into a category of activities collectively known as 'activities of daily living' (ADLs). These include personal hygiene and grooming, dressing and undressing, self-feeding, functional transfers, bowel and bladder management and ambulation. Personal hygiene and grooming is of vital importance to the health and wellbeing of the person with dementia. The stage to which the dementia has progressed will influence whether dressing and bathing is an issue for the carer and the person with dementia.

In the early stages, the person may want to continue to be groomed and bathed as they would normally; the regularity and familiarity of these actions may provide structure for the person with dementia and maintenance of routine can be a source of comfort for them. The carer may use this routine to assist the person with dementia to regulate their day. Stokes (2010) gives practical advice on ways to cope with everyday life and dementia. His suggestions include encouraging the person to continue with everyday activities, keeping tasks short and interesting, laying out the person's clothes and watching for signs of the need for toileting like fidgeting and pulling at clothes.

As the disease progresses the person with dementia may begin to lose interest in their hygiene or appearance. They will experience diminishing cognition and over time their abilities will decline and it can be expected that total dependence will eventuate. The challenge for the carer is to help them maintain independence as much as possible, for as long as possible (Alzheimer's Australia, 2000).

The task-like nature of hygiene and grooming permits the carer to break down the activity into steps. This process can make more complex tasks easier for a person with dementia. In this way the person may be able to continue many personal hygiene and grooming tasks even when the disease has progressed.

The level of support required from the carer will range from prompting and supporting, to full completion of all tasks as the person with dementia progressively loses their independence. It is important to identify what the specific steps in the individual's personal hygiene and grooming routine actually are. In doing so, it is possible to focus on those steps that they can continue to perform. Maintaining a sense of independence is positive for both the carer and the person with dementia. Focusing on what the person with dementia can do for themselves and only providing assistance for the tasks that they struggle with can help maintain independence as well as promote self-esteem. Sidani, Streiner and LeClerc (2011) argue that an abilities-focused approach can positively assist people with dementia to participate in the care they require at the start of their day. The need for carer intervention will also be influenced significantly by the continence status of the person with dementia. If the person is unaware of their level of continence then the need for personal hygiene and redressing during the course of the day may become more and more frequent. Incontinence is a significant factor in the need for residential care (Frederick & Turton, 2006). (Strategies that can assist carers to manage incontinence are discussed in more detail in Chapter 5.)

The tasks required for personal hygiene and grooming include bathing, hair care and styling, shaving, oral care, skin care, nail care, ear and eye care (Alzheimer's Australia, 2005). The carer may be required to assist with some or all of these tasks and the person with dementia may respond differently to any of them depending on their past life experience and the stage of their disease.

This chapter aims to outline how both paid and unpaid family carers within the residential or community setting can assess and respond to the personal hygiene and grooming needs of the person with dementia. The two main tasks of personal hygiene and grooming are dressing and bathing and these are discussed next.

Dressing

The task of dressing includes clothing selection, undressing and redressing as well as the use of make-up. It is important to engage the person with dementia in decision-making as much as possible. Showing them what clothes are available and helping them choose what they wear is important. This will not always be the case but will be important in the early stages. Offering a choice between two items can be less overwhelming while still promoting independence and self esteem. The type of clothing may also be significant depending on how dependent the person is. Loose fitting and buttoned or zipped clothing may be the easiest to deal with. Several companies manufacture clothing specifically for people with dementia; these types of clothes are often referred to as 'adaptive clothing'. Enclosed supportive shoes with velcro instead of laces are also important in maintaining balance and protecting feet from injury. The use of a shoehorn may also be beneficial.

When laying out clothes place them in the order in which they are applied. For example, place underwear first, followed by socks, a shirt and trousers, then shoes. This will prompt the person with dementia and may assist in maintaining a level of independence.

As dementia progresses it can become increasingly difficult for the person to dress independently. Providing one item of clothing at a time can assist the person to complete the task. Keeping a calm quiet environment and reducing distractions can also assist the person with dementia to focus on what they are doing.

If the person has a deficit in their ability to move their arms or legs, undressing and redressing can become an issue. In this case, the good arm or leg is undressed first and when redressing the affected arm or leg is attended first. If incontinence is an issue the use of commercially available incontinence pads is advised.

Application of make-up may continue to be important for some women as this can make them feel attractive (Villafranca, Dougherty & Lindstrom, 2011); however, it is advisable to keep this to a minimum. A lipstick may be all that is necessary and complex make up like eye shadow or eyeliner is best avoided, within the person's tolerance.

Bathing

Remaining clean is of vital importance to skin integrity. Regular cleaning of the skin reduces the incidence of skin irritation, rashes and dryness, which can cause the skin to break down resulting in the development of a wound or pressure sore. The frequency of bathing will depend on the person's level of activity and whether they are experiencing incontinence. Daily bathing or showering will not automatically be necessary. Bathing can become difficult for some people with dementia due to factors such as pain, fatigue and weakness, fear, anxiety and discomfort (Rader et al., 2006). In these cases, it is important to address the problems whilst also maintaining hygiene. The carers' actions should aim to provide comfort, safety and relaxation. As mentioned previously, to help maintain the person with dementia's independence, it may be helpful to break tasks down into steps. They may be able to continue bathing tasks, such as washing their face or cleaning their teeth, even when the disease is well established.

Don't rush or be forceful when bathing the person with dementia as this will cause confusion and resistance. Hoeffer et al. (2006) report that in previous studies 'aggressive behaviour often was displayed in response to a caregiver demand during personal care and subsided when the interaction was ceased' (p. 525). If you encounter resistance distract the person or leave them for a short period and return and try again. Remain calm and gentle, speak softly and reassure them that everything is alright, communicate what is happening and what the next step will be.

The person with dementia may at certain times be resistant to any form of showering or bathing. This could be due to feeling powerless, out of control or frightened (Sloane et al., 2004). It is important to remember that when a person with dementia becomes agitated or resistant they are trying to communicate that something is upsetting them. Stopping or altering the activity can often relieve the agitation (Johnson, 2011). This may mean that the whole task of bathing is not completed each time. However, by concentrating on the person, not the task of bathing, the chances of a successful experience are increased. Sloane et al. (2004) found that resistiveness and agitation during bathing can be reduced by as much as 60% by adopting a person-centred approach. If the person with dementia has become resistive to bathing consider a wash over a basin instead or offer a wet washer after they have used the toilet. No-rinse soaps are useful if the person with dementia can only tolerate a short bathing experience. Having a range of strategies can help ensure that the bathing experience is more relaxing and enjoyable for both the person with dementia and their carers. Further information and strategies for behaviours that are causing concern can be found in Chapter 7.

Try and establish a routine so that the person with dementia becomes used to attending to hygiene at a given time of the day. For example, tell the person it is time for their bath and prepare the bathroom. You may need to turn the heating on, close the windows, have the towels, shampoo and soap ready and lay out their clothes. If a plunge bath is the preferred option drawing the bath in readiness and testing the temperature will avoid delays once the person with dementia is in the room. Plunge baths may, however, prove difficult to get into and out of (there are commercially available lifters for this) and for this reason a shower with a suitable shower chair may be preferred. A hand–held shower hose (which can be easily retro-fitted) is also useful as this can be easily directed at various parts of the body.

Bathroom safety is vital; the person with dementia needs to feel secure and the carer needs the assurance that the person will not fall. The installation of grab rails near the shower or bath and toilet, along with anti–slip mats, is recommended. These items can be obtained from local Independent Living Centres (Alzheimer's Australia, 2005). Stokes (2010) also recommends the installation of a thermostatic mixing valve to avoid the possibility of scalding.

When undressing the person with dementia, maintain their privacy, dignity and comfort and ensure the room is warm and private. Forewarn the person of what is happening and avoid pulling clothes off. Have them sit down to remove shoes, socks, skirts, trousers and underwear, and quickly and gently remove clothes over the head. If undressing in another room ensure the person is wearing a dressing gown or other suitable covering when walking between the room and the bathroom. If undressing causes distress leave areas covered with towels or even partly dressed and work around them.

Once in the bathroom test the temperature of the water before applying to the skin and ask the person to feel the water by pouring it gently on their hand. Avoid spraying water over the body or the head without first ensuring the person is prepared, as this may cause a negative reaction and some people may even lash out at the carer.

Work quickly, but carefully, from head to toe. Wet a face cloth and give it to the person. They may use it to wash their own face or they may simply hold it while the carer performs the task.

Other hygiene needs

Hair care

If shampooing is necessary, wet the hair, apply the shampoo and leave it in whilst performing another task. Non-irritating shampoos, such as a baby shampoo, are recommended, as they will not sting if they accidentally come in contact with the eyes. When rinsing the hair, forewarn the person and have them close their eyes. If medicated shampoos are used tilt the head backwards and rinse from the front. Using a brush to rinse the water through the hair may also prove effective.

Depending on personal preference, many people with dementia may get pleasure from regular visits to the hairdresser; this should be encouraged. It is recommended that hair is keep short for ease of care and to avoid knotting.

Body washing

Many people do not use soap on their face, so its use is best avoided to prevent irritation to the eyes. Establish the person's preference in this area before commencing. To begin, wash the person's face with a face washer. Using a second face washer with soap, start at the shoulders and neck (this may be an opportunity to give the person a gentle massage) and work your way down the body, paying attention to the underarms and hands. Next, wash the back and then the chest, rinsing as you go. For women, pay particular attention to the area under the breasts, ensuring that no soap is left, as this may cause irritation and even skin breakdown. Following this, wash the legs and feet including between the toes. Finally, using a different face washer, wash the genital area front to back. This is particularly important for people who are incontinent. When choosing a soap use one that is non-drying with a neutral pH. Those containing sodium laurel sulphate can be very drying. Liquid soaps can also be very effective. A discussion about what type of soap to use with the person's doctor or nurse may be of benefit.

Bed bathing

As the person's mobility decreases (or as a practical alternative to showering), bed bathing may become necessary. Rader et al. (2006) argue that a bed bath with a warm towel may help reduce behavioural symptoms by as much as 38% and also assist in reducing skin dryness. To perform a bed bath you will require a suitable bowl for water, towels and face washers. Commercially available 'bath-in-a-bag' products may also be used for this purpose. Begin with water at body temperature and after removing the person's clothing, cover their body with towels; this will help maintain warmth, privacy and dignity. Using a wet face washer, start at the face, then soap the washer and clean the hands, next move to the arms and underarms. Allowing the person to drape their hands into the water bowl may prove comforting and more effectively clean the hands. Rolling the person from side to side or, if able, sitting the person up, wash the shoulders and the back, drying the skin as you go (leave the towel in place to cover). Next move to the legs and feet and ensure you wash and dry between the toes. If necessary, refresh and warm the water as you go. Lastly, clean and dry the genital area, paying particular attention if the person is incontinent.

Drying

Soft fluffy towels are recommended for drying as they are less abrasive on the skin. Begin by drying the hair, head and the face. For people with long hair, a hair dryer may be necessary after the rest of the body has been dried. Next, using a second towel in the same sequence as washing, dry the arms, shoulders, back, chest (ensuring that the area under breasts is dry), legs, feet (ensuring the area between the toes is dry) and finally the genital area.

Once dry, apply a personal deodorant. You may find a roll-on most suitable as spray cans may cause distress if the purpose is unclear to the person. A perfume may also be applied if desired; however, this may lead to skin dryness, rash or irritation so discontinue if this occurs. Dryness can cause skin to break down so finishing off with the application of a skin cream, such as sorbolene, may prove successful in maintaining flexibility and decrease fragility.

Shaving

Electric razors are recommended for safety reasons; however, a safety razor blade may be used with care. Using shaving foam and holding the skin taught will give the best results and will avoid nicks and cuts. For women, shaving underarms and legs may be important. If so, using a safety razor whilst in the shower may be best.

Oral care

Due to potential neglect, the person with dementia will be susceptible to oral diseases such as gingivitis, plaque build-up, dry mouth, thrush and stomatitis. Good oral hygiene and dental care is therefore essential. Teeth brushing is recommended after bathing; however, gaining cooperation may be an issue. The use of a mild toothpaste and a small, soft children's toothbrush may prove successful. An electric toothbrush may also be tried, within the person's tolerance (Villafranca et al., 2011). To begin this process, give them the toothbrush with the paste on it; depending on their ability they may brush themselves. If not, stand in front of them and encourage them to open their mouth, gently brushing the surface of each tooth. Holding the brush at a 45-degree angle to the gum line, brush the outer, inner and chewing surfaces of the teeth using small circular motions. Break up the mouth into quadrants, and work through each section, allowing the person to spit between quadrants. If they are uncooperative, regular mouth rinsing with water or mouthwashes during the day may also prove useful. A regular dental check for these people is recommended. For people with dentures, a clean with a toothbrush or nailbrush may be all that is necessary, whilst some people rely on denture soakers.

The South Australian Dental Service (2009) recommends that those with dementia:

▶ brush morning and night

- ▶ use a high fluoride toothpaste
- ▶ use a soft toothbrush applied to gums, tongue and teeth
- ▶ use an antibacterial mouthwash after lunch
- ▶ keep their mouth moist
- ▶ reduce their intake of sugar-rich foods.

Nail care

Fingernails and toenails should be inspected at each bath time. While bathing the person with dementia, clean under their nails with a soft nailbrush. Keep nails clipped and short (using safety clippers) to avoid scratching and skin tears. The frequency of clipping will depend on the individual's nail growth, but fingernail clipping once a week and toe nail clipping every four to six weeks is not unusual. Nail buffing is also recommended. For some people manicures and pedicures are a source of comfort. A podiatrist may be necessary for some people, particularly those with diabetes. Paid carers should ensure that they follow their organisation's policy in relation to cutting fingernails and toenails.

Ear care

The inside of the ears are self-cleaning; however, a build-up of cerumen (ear wax) can lead to hearing difficulties. If this occurs consult the person's doctor. Cleaning the outer ear with a damp face washer is generally all that will be required. Gently wipe over the surface and clean into the folds and the back of the ears.

Eye care

The eyes will not require any special cleaning; however, the use of a damp face washer or a damp tissue may be necessary to remove any build-up of eye secretions (sleep). If this is the case, gently wipe the eyes from the lids downward, over the lashes and from the nose to the ear in a single movement. Use a separate section of the washer for each eye.

Practical advice and tips

Dressing

A summary of the practical tips for dressing is listed below. If possible, carers should:

- recommend using adaptive clothing and/or velcro 'laced' shoes
- undress the person's good arm or leg first and when redressing start with the affected arm or leg first
- break down tasks into smaller more manageable steps
- use commercially available incontinence pads.

Bathing

A summary of the practical tips for bathing is listed below. If possible, carers should:

- try to maintain the person's independence as much as possible
- adopt a calm, flexible and person-centred approach
- break down tasks into smaller more manageable steps
- maintain safety, ensure privacy and use a skin-appropriate soap and eye-safe shampoo
- consider using bed bathing; daily bathing or showering may not be necessary in some instances (Costello & Corcoran, 2009)
- look for breaks in the skin whilst conducting the bathing routine and ensure the skin is dry after bathing to avoid skin breakdown.

Conclusion

Personal hygiene and grooming are essential for the wellbeing of a person with dementia. The carer plays a vital role in this and can assist in maintaining independence by allowing them to do things for themselves as much as possible. If behaviours develop around the need for grooming and personal hygiene the carer may need to address these through investigating and understanding the causes of the behaviours. Assistance in developing appropriate strategies may need to be sought from a healthcare professional. Grooming and personal hygiene also presents an ideal opportunity for the carer to review the person for skin breakdown, which can lead to the development of a wound that may require referral to a healthcare professional.

References

Alzheimer's Australia. (2000). *Help sheet 39: The bathroom and toilet.* Melbourne: Alzheimer's Australia.

Alzheimer's Australia. (2005). *Help sheet 17: Hygiene.* Melbourne: Alzheimer's Australia.

Costello, E., & Corcoran, M. A. (2009). Bathing individuals with dementia: An evidence based review of current practice. *Geriatrics and Aging, 12*(9), 464–468.

Frederick, J., & Turton, J. (2006). *A continence service for older people.* Canberra: Department of Health & Ageing, Victorian Government.

Hoeffer, B., Talerico, K. A., Rasin, J., Mitchell, C. M., Stewart, B. J., McKenzie, D., Barrick, A. L., Rader, J., & Sloane, P. D. (2006). Assisting cognitively impaired nursing home residents with bathing: Effects of two bathing interventions on caregiving. *The Gerontologist, 46*(4), 524–532.

Johnson, R. H. (2011). Practical care: Creative strategies for bathing. *Nursing and Residential Care, 13*(8), 392–394.

Rader, J., Barrick, A. L., Hoeffer, B., Sloane, P. D., McKenzie, D., Talerico, K. A., & Glover, J. U. (2006). The bathing of older adults with dementia: Easing the unnecessarily unpleasant aspects of assisted bathing. *American Journal of Nursing, 106*(4), 40–48.

Sidani, S., Streiner, D., & LeClerc, C. (2011). Evaluating the effectiveness of the abilities-focused approach to morning care of people with dementia. *International Journal of Older People Nursing, 7*(1), 37–45. doi: 10.111/j.1748-3743.2011.00273.x

Sloane, P. D., Hoeffer, B., Mitchell, C. M., McKenzie, D. A., Barrick, A. L., Rader, J., Stewart, B. J., Talerico, K. A., Rasin, J. A., Zink, R. C., & Koch, G. G. (2004). Effects of person-centred showering and the towel bath on bathing-associated aggression, agitation and discomfort in nursing home residents with dementia: A randomised controlled trial. *Journal of American Geriatrics Society, 52*(11), 1795–1804.

South Australian Dental Service. (2009). *Better oral health in residential care.* Retrieved from http://www.health.gov.au/internet/main/publishing.nsf/Content/2DC945BED2046270CA25760E001E8B2E/$File/FacilitatorPortfolio.pdf

Stokes, G. (2010). Explaining about day to day living with dementia. *Working with Older People, 14*(1), 5–7. doi: 10.5042/wwop.2010.0070

Villafranca, V., Dougherty, J., & Lindstrom, K. B. (2011). Dressing and grooming. In G.A. Martin & M. N. Sabbagh (Eds.), *Palliative care for advanced Alzheimer's and dementia: Guidelines and standards for evidence-based care.* New York: Springer Publishing Co.

Chapter 3

EATING AND SWALLOWING

Shyama G K Ratnayake
University of Western Sydney

Suzanne Brownhill
University of Western Sydney

Chapter outcomes

When you have completed this chapter you will be able to:

- take a holistic approach to feeding
- maximise mealtimes and encourage independence
- manage mealtime difficulties.

Keywords

dementia, eating difficulties, swallowing difficulties, nutritional intake, feeding assistance, carers

Introduction

People with dementia may experience a change in personality and impaired social function. At the onset of the disease, individuals may show signs of having difficulty with activities of daily living (ADLs) and as the disease progresses any mental and physical problems may become severe. Feeding and the ability to swallow is the last activity of daily living to deteriorate. Even though people in the early stages of dementia have an increased appetite (hyperphagia), difficulty with eating and swallowing (which, as the disease progresses, can lead to weight loss and undernutrition) will become increasingly evident (Amella, 2008; Chang & Roberts, 2008; Keller, Edward & Cook, 2007).

What are the risks of undernutrition and weight loss?

Those who experience eating and swallowing difficulty at meal times are at higher risk of undernutrition and dehydration. Risk of undernutrition and weight loss is higher in people with dementia due to their age and other illnesses such as heart failure, kidney failure, lung conditions and depression. Dehydration and muscle wasting may lead to skin breakdown (e.g. pressure sores and ulcers) in people with dementia and a decreased resistance to disease may make them more vulnerable to infection. These can increase the risk of illness (morbidity) and death (mortality) (Alzheimer's Australia, 2009; Palliative Care Dementia Interface, 2011).

What are the nutritional requirements of people with dementia?

The nutritional requirements of people with dementia are the same as for other older people; all need a balanced diet. With less physical activity, fewer calories are required but there is a greater need for vitamins, minerals, fibre and fluids. A diet consisting mainly of vegetables, fruits, legumes, cereals, moderate amounts of fish and dairy products (which contain high levels of monounsaturated fatty acids), Vitamins B12 and folate, as well as antioxidants (including Vitamin E, carotenoids and flavonoids) can be beneficial. To reduce saturated fat levels, low consumption of meat and poultry is also recommended (Féart et al., 2009).

Fluids help to protect against infection and help to maintain skin integrity and general good health. Low fluid intake and dehydration is often a problem for people with dementia, so they should always have access to fluids and be encouraged to drink.

Mealtime difficulties

Mealtimes are opportunities for family gatherings, social connection and a source of enjoyment. Food, and the eating of it, constitutes every culture. Food is almost always shared and is a gesture of love, generosity and caring. Therefore, the inability to feed or to share a meal with a loved one can be a frustrating experience. Family members and carers of people with dementia can face this situation daily. Mealtime capabilities and difficulties will vary depending on the person's stage of illness.

What are the manifestations of mealtime difficulties?

As progression and manifestations of dementia varies from one person to another, it is often hard to anticipate difficulties that may occur at each mealtime. It follows that it is hard to know how to manage those difficulties. In the early stages of dementia, people will show some signs of memory loss, cognitive impairment or lack of motor control, mood changes, anxiety and a loss of spontaneity and motivation. These difficulties and impairments will become evident in their daily activities. For example, confusion and poor concentration and attention are likely to affect their ability to feed themselves. When difficulties in eating and swallowing occur, encouragement and regular assistance with verbal cues will be required. Examples of verbal cues include: 'That sandwich looks good' or 'It is nice to eat together, isn't it?'

As the disease progresses, their dependence on others at mealtimes will increase, as will the need for closer monitoring and greater assistance. Examples of mealtime issues may include:

▶ wandering
▶ spitting out food
▶ refusing food
▶ rejecting food put in the mouth
▶ restlessness and agitation

- difficulty in effectively getting food into the mouth
- difficulty in recognising eating utensils and food.

In late stage dementia, people need constant supervision and full assistance with feeding as they may have swallowing issues (dysphagia) (Alzheimer's Australia, 2009; Keller et al., 2007; Palliative Care Dementia Interface, 2011).

What factors contribute to mealtime difficulties?

Mealtimes focus on nutritional intake and hydration. There are a number of factors that can make that process difficult for people with dementia. Contributory factors include:

- **thinking (cognitive) impairment,** which is a major sign and symptom associated with dementia – people with dementia who have an impaired memory may not be able to recognise food or know what to do with it
- **physical dysfunction** that is related to feeding and includes the loss of small movements of the fingers (fine motor skills) required by the action of self-feeding. It also includes the loss of the ability to use eating utensils due to apraxia: the impaired ability to perform skilled or purposeful movements
- **psychological (mental) issues,** particularly depression. Symptoms of depression include loss of appetite, lethargy, slower movements and impaired concentration, which are all likely to hinder nutritional and fluid intake and make feeding difficult. Agitation and aggression may also become more evident in the middle and later stages of dementia and may result in a lowered intake of food and fluid due to refusal of food and assistance
- **social isolation** due to psychological, interpersonal or environmental reasons, which can cause mealtimes to be unappealing and mundane
- **environments** that are distracting and stressful – these can interfere with fluid and food intake
- **cultural attributes** that can influence food and fluid intake at meal times. (British Geriatrics Society, 2009; Chang & Roberts, 2008; Korczyn & Halperin, 2009; Mamhidir et al., 2007; Palliative Care Dementia Interface, 2011; Simmons et al., 2008).

How to manage mealtime difficulties

Dementia can present certain difficulties during mealtime, both for the person being assisted and the person assisting. A number of challenges and changes require adjustment on the part of caregivers (Keller et al., 2007). Possible strategies and adaptations that may be implemented during mealtimes include:

▶ delivering an individualised approach to meals, including a choice of food, timing and pacing of assistance

▶ being aware of gradual (or not so gradual) 'out of character' behavioural changes that impede or hinder nutritional intake (e.g. agitation may occur when a mealtime routine is broken or when a person's health status changes)

▶ checking for physical problems that may be a barrier to nutritional intake (e.g. dental problems)

▶ ensuring appropriate oral care is given

▶ checking the psychological wellbeing of the person with dementia (accompanying co-morbid conditions, such as depression and anxiety, may require professional assessment and help)

▶ considering the cultural background and food preferences of the person with dementia

▶ ensuring the position of the one assisting with feeding is seated at the same level as the person being fed – face-to-face positioning and eye contact improves social engagement and interaction and allows for direct observation of any probelms that might arise

▶ being aware of, and if possible changing, any environmental aspects that hinder or distract from the mealtime and nutritional intake – choose an environment in which eating and drinking may be enjoyed

▶ minimising environmental noise and the level of distraction from television and music – this will enhance and encourage personal conversation and interaction between the person being assisted with feeding and the caregiver

▶ optimising mealtimes to maximise the benefits nutritionally, physically and relationally (allowing at least 30 minutes) – rushing food intake can cause choking and aspiration and lead to serious problems such as pneumonia

- prompting and encouraging people with dementia with words or gestures to eat and drink
- encouraging mealtimes and the consumption of food and fluid in the dining room, rather than in bed or in a wheelchair
- selecting music preferred by the person being assisted with eating and drinking
- ensuring the lighting is adequate and is not producing glare or shadow
- stimulating the appetite by preparing and serving food that is visually appealing and pleasant to smell in an area adjacent to or in the dining area
- using appropriate utensils, for example, soft spoons (an occupational therapist can assist in evaluating feeding and drinking requirements) (Amella, 2008; Alzheimer's Australia, 2009; Keller et al., 2007; Layne, 1990; Palliative Care Dementia Interface, 2011).

Families can experience difficulties when they eat out with a family member with dementia. However, careful planning and adopting practical strategies to suit the occasion will resolve most of the problems (Keller et al., 2007). For instance, families could:

- choose a quieter restaurant and go during a slower time of the day in terms of customer flow
- sit in a quieter area of the restaurant
- provide the person with simple menu choices
- sit close to the person to assist them with eating and drinking.

Weight loss and the inability to swallow are common problems among people with severe and end stage dementia. In these situations, which can be distressing for carers, consultation with, and support of, health professionals is essential.

Maximising mealtime: encouraging independence

Most of us enjoy a certain level of independence. It therefore follows that the person who is being fed needs to maintain their own independence for as long as possible. Think of subtle or discrete ways that can facilitate or foster their independence. For example, cut up their food, leave out nutritional snacks and serve foods that are easy to handle and ready-to-eat (e.g. peeled fruits cut into small pieces).

If possible, join in and eat at the same time as the person you are assisting. For example, you could share nutritional finger food, which promotes conversation and interaction.

When and where possible allow the person the opportunity to make their own decisions about what, how and where they would prefer to eat and drink. Gauge the level of assistance they need to maintain their independence.

Swallowing difficulties and aspirated pneumonia

Swallowing is a complex process that involves the mouth, tongue, pharynx and oesophagus. Swallowing difficulties (dysphagia) are common among people with severe and end stage dementia. In this situation, fluids and food may pass into the airway instead of down the oesophagus. Aspirated food and liquid in the lungs can cause pneumonia (aspirated pneumonia) and its complications can be fatal (Layne, 1990). Possible signs of swallowing difficulties (dysphagia) include:

▶ a gurgling voice after swallowing
▶ coughing during or after eating
▶ prolonged chewing
▶ regurgitation of food through the mouth or nose
▶ pooling of food in the mouth
▶ extensive chewing without swallowing (pouching)
▶ excessive drooling
▶ recurrent chest infections (Layne, 1990).

Management of dysphagia

If dysphagia is suspected, it is important to refer the person with dementia to a speech pathologist. A speech pathologist can assess the person and recommend suitable and helpful strategies to manage the dysphagia. Usually compensatory strategies, such as postural techniques and modification of diet, are recommended. A guideline of correct and individualised feeding techniques and strategies can then be implemented (Layne, 1990).

Postural techniques

Positioning is important while feeding. The person being assisted to eat and swallow should be in a 60- to 90-degree upright position with the head flexed forward. The person who is assisting with feeding should sit at or below eye level. A relaxed and socially amenable environment with minimal distraction can also help to focus on the eating and swallowing process.

Once positioned, small amounts of food should be offered to the person and they should be fed slowly, allowing rest periods in between. The recommended average time to promote adequate oral intake is between 35 and 40 minutes (Layne, 1990). Orientation to mealtime and use of appropriate verbal cueing also encourages eating. For example, 'We are going to have lunch' or 'Swallow the food in your mouth'.

Dietary modifications

Thin fluids (all regular liquids with low viscosity) are difficult to control in the mouth and can easily and quickly go down the airway. A speech pathologist can assess the person's capabilities and recommend the appropriate texture of food and viscosity of fluids. Fluids need to be thickened using thickeners to the appropriate consistency; for example, nectar, honey and pudding-thick liquids (Layne, 1990). A textured diet with food soft enough to mash is usually recommended in the case of moderate swallowing difficulty and pureed food in severe swallowing difficulty. Dry and crumbly foods as well as sticky foods need to be avoided as they will exacerbate impaired swallowing.

Oral hygiene and dental care

Taking care of the mouth is important in maintaining good nutrition in dementia as problems arising from gum and teeth and dentures can cause loss of appetite. See Chapter 2 on personal hygiene and grooming.

Conclusion

This chapter was aimed at helping carers to manage or avert feeding and swallowing difficulties. It invites carers to take a holistic approach to feeding or assisting with feeding, to maximise mealtimes, manage mealtime difficulties and to promote independence of the person being assisted.

References

Alzheimer's Australia. (2009). *Caring for someone with dementia*. Retrieved from http://www.fightdementia.org.au/understanding-dementia/section-2-caring-for-someone-with-dementia.aspx

Amella, E. J. (2008). Mealtime difficulties. In E. Capezuti, D. Zwicker, M. Mezey & T. Fulmer (Eds.), *Evidence-based geriatric nursing protocols for best practice* (3rd ed., pp. 337–351). New York: Springer Publishing Co.

British Geriatrics Society. (2009). *Good practice guides: Nutritional advice in common clinical situations* [web page]. Retrieved from http://www.bgs.org.uk/index.php?option=com_content&view=article&id=41:gpgnutrition&catid=12:goodpractice&Itemid=106

Chang, C.-C., & Roberts, B. L. (2008). Feeding difficulty in older adults with dementia. *Journal of Clinical Nursing, 17*(17), 2266–2274. doi: 10.1111/j.1365-2702.2007.02275.x

Féart, C., Samieri, C., Rondeau, V., Amieva, H., Portet, F., Dartigues, J. F., Barberger-Gataua, P., & Scarmeas, N. (2009). Adherence to a Mediterranean diet, cognitive decline, and risk of dementia. *The Journal of the American Medical Association, 302*(6), 638-648. doi:10.1001/jama.2009.1146

Keller, H. H., Edward, G., & Cook, C. (2007). Mealtime experiences of families with dementia. *American Journal of Alzheimer's Disease & Other Dementia, 21*(6), 431–438.

Korczyn, A. D., & Halperin, I. (2009). Depression and dementia. *Journal of the Neurological Sciences, 283*(1–2), 139–142. doi: 10.1016/j.jns.2009.02.346

Layne, K. (1990). Feeding strategies for dysphagic patient: A nursing perspective. *Dysphagia, 5,* 84–88.

Mamhidir, A.-G., Karlsson, I., Norberg, A., & Mona, K. (2007). Weight increase in patients with dementia, and alteration in meal routines and meal environment after integrity promoting care. *Journal of Clinical Nursing, 16*(5), 987–996. doi: 10.1111/j.1365-2702.2006.01780.x

Palliative Care Dementia Interface: Enhancing Community Capacity Project. (2011). *Dementia: Information for families and friends of people with severe and end stage dementia* (3rd ed.). Sydney: University of Western Sydney.

Simmons, S. F., Keeler, E., Zhuo, X., Hickey, K. A., Sato, H.-W., & Schnelle, J. F. (2008). Prevention of unintentional weight loss in nursing home residents: A controlled trial of feeding assistance. *Journal of the American Geriatrics Society, 56*(8), 1466–1473. doi: 10.1111/j.1532-5415.2008.01801.x

Chapter 4

PROMOTING SLEEP

Deborah Hatcher
University of Western Sydney

Kathleen Dixon
University of Western Sydney

Chapter outcomes

When you have completed this chapter you will be able to:

▶ describe the stages of sleep

▶ understand how dementia affects sleep

▶ use strategies to improve sleep and manage sleep disturbance for the person who has dementia.

Keywords

sleep, sleep disturbance, dementia, older people, carer

Introduction

Sleep is important for health and wellbeing. It is a calm period in which body systems are able to rest, restore energy and repair tissue damage. It is also an important time for the brain to make new pathways for information processing and to store into memory information gained throughout the day (Porth, 2011). We all need a good night's sleep; however, our need for sleep and our patterns of sleep change as we age and this can lead to sleep disturbance. Those of us who have experienced sleepless nights know about the subsequent impact on our ability to function the next day. For a person with dementia, disturbed sleep patterns can cause problems not only for themselves but also for their carers.

This chapter will present an overview of sleep, summarising the stages of sleep and the disruptions to sleep relating to ageing and dementia. It will describe common causes of sleep disturbance, as well as strategies to assist you in managing these disturbances and promoting sleep for the person with dementia. It will highlight the importance of a good night's sleep to enhance the safety, health and wellbeing of the person with dementia and your ability to provide care for them.

Stages of sleep

Sleep is categorised into two stages known as rapid eye movement sleep or REM sleep and non-rapid eye movement sleep or non-REM sleep (Eeles, 2006; Holland et al., 2008). Understanding the different stages of sleep has been made possible by the study of brain waves through the use of an instrument known as an electroencephalogram (EEG). The EEG (which is a very similar instrument to the electrocardiogram or ECG) is used to measure the frequency and amplitude of brain waves. The types of brain waves that occur during sleep are called delta and theta waves and it is the presence of these slower wave patterns that tell us that most of our brain cells are not very active and we are in fact asleep. Brain waves are affected by a number of things including ageing, disease states (in particular, brain diseases) and chemical and sensory stimuli (Marieb, 2012).

When we first become drowsy we experience non-REM sleep, which consists of four stages, with each stage representing an increasing depth of sleep. Stage 1 is a brief stage of one to seven minutes duration. It occurs at the onset of sleep and acts as the transition from wakefulness to sleep. During this stage it is fairly easy to rouse the sleeping person by simply calling their name. Stage 2 is a deeper period of sleep, lasting somewhere between 10 and 25 minutes. Stage 3 is a short period of deep sleep that leads into Stage 4, which is a more prolonged period of deep sleep lasting between 20 and 40 minutes. It is during this last phase, when we are deeply asleep, that our muscles are relaxed (although we intermittently adjust our posture) and we experience a lowering of blood pressure, heart rate and gastrointestinal activity. It is much more difficult to be roused from sleep during Stage 4 than it is at the onset of sleep. It is during Stages 3 and 4 that we are most likely to experience nightmares (Marieb, 2012; Porth, 2011).

About 90 minutes after the onset of sleep we experience REM sleep. During this period of sleep, our eye movements are rapid, the brain replays memories and we have vivid dreams. There is also a loss of muscle movement and tone, akin to a temporary paralysis, which is thought to protect us from responding in a physical way to our dreams. During REM sleep the brain uses a great deal of oxygen, so in order to meet this demand there is an increase in heart rate, blood pressure, breathing and body temperature (Marieb, 2012; Porth, 2011). During any one night we might experience four to six periods of REM sleep (Lehne, 2010).

Ageing and sleep

It is thought that sleep is important because in non-REM sleep the brain and other body systems are able to rest and during REM sleep the brain is able to process and store into memory events that happened during the day, as well as eliminate unimportant things from memory (Marieb, 2012). As we age, there is an increased likelihood that the quality and quantity of sleep will be impaired. This is because older people tend to have more disrupted sleep and experience shorter or non-existent Stages 3 and 4. Compared to younger people, older people take longer to fall asleep, have more awakenings during the night and wake earlier in the morning. These changes to sleep patterns can have serious consequences for health and wellbeing, leading to a decrease in quality of life, an increase in risk of falls and accidents and, where breathing is impaired during sleep, such as during snoring or sleep apnoea, these changes can have a deleterious effect on the heart, lungs and brain (Porth, 2011).

Studies have demonstrated that sleep is important for maintaining cognitive functioning and lack of sleep has a negative impact on cognition (Waters & Bucks, 2011). For people with dementia, in addition to sleep disturbances caused by ageing, sleep can be further disrupted by increasing levels of confusion and delirium and a tendency to wander at night (Gabelle & Dauvilliers, 2010; Porth, 2011). Disruption to sleep can also lead to increased impairment of physical and mental function in people with dementia and can cause distress and depression in both the person and their carers (Ancoli-Israel & Vitiello, 2006; Gabelle & Dauvilliers, 2010; Lee & Thomas, 2011). Sleep disruption has also been associated with an increase in mortality (Martin et al., 2006).

Strategies for managing sleep disturbance

Managing sleep disturbance in the person with dementia can be challenging and requires a multifaceted approach (Eeles, 2006). It is essential to find the cause of the problem as this will influence the strategies you use to promote sleep, assist in maintaining living at home and delay transfer to other care settings (Ancoli-Israel & Vitiello, 2006; Eeles, 2006; Lee & Thomas, 2011). The causes of sleep disturbance are complex and can be broadly categorised under physical, psychological, environmental and socio-cultural factors. The second part of this chapter describes these factors and provides suggestions to promote sleep for the person with dementia.

Physical factors

Physical factors disrupting sleep are those related to the anatomy and physiology of the body (Holland et al., 2008). These include damage to the brain caused by dementia, resulting in an inability to differentiate between day and night; acute illnesses, such as a cold or urinary tract infection; the presence of chronic conditions, for example, diabetes or depression; pain from conditions such as arthritis; side effects of medications; hunger or thirst; and incontinence.

Strategies to deal with physical factors that disrupt sleep

Strategies that address these physical causes and minimise disruption to sleep are listed below. Carers should:

▶ consult a doctor for diagnosis and management of medical conditions

▶ organise regular check-ups to manage chronic conditions

▶ give adequate pain relief (in consultation with a doctor)

▶ check to see if sleep disruption is a side effect of medication or over-the-counter drugs, as these can sometimes interfere with sleep

▶ discuss with a doctor the possibility of prescribing medication to help the person sleep (sometimes this is useful as a short-term strategy to establish a sleep pattern; however, there needs to be careful consideration in using this approach as research has shown the use of sedatives have been associated with increased falls, hospitalisation and mortality)

▶ offer a snack, herbal tea or warm milk before bedtime or during the night if the person wakes

▶ avoid giving a large meal before bedtime

▶ encourage a warm shower or bath before bedtime

▶ assist the person to the toilet before bedtime

▶ try to help the person into their preferred sleeping position.

Psychological factors

Psychological factors also compromise sleep and these relate to intellectual functioning and previous experiences and behaviours (Holland et al., 2008). They include sleeping during the day (Ancoli–Israel & Vitiello, 2006; Martin et al., 2006); going to bed early; confusion and disorientation at the end of the day due to decreased sensory ability and sensory stimulation (referred to as sundowning) (Harris, Nagy & Vardaxis, 2009); evening agitation; inadequate exercise or activity during the day (Holland et al., 2008; Lee & Thomas, 2011); consuming caffeine or alcohol; smoking; feeling lost or frightened; and dreaming.

Strategies to deal with psychological factors that disrupt sleep

Strategies to address these psychological causes and minimise disruption to sleep are listed below. Carers should:

▶ maintain a daily routine
▶ find out the person's usual sleep patterns, including quantity and quality of sleep
▶ prevent sleeping in the daytime (except for a rest after lunch)
▶ promote daily exposure to the sun, as exposure to natural bright light has been found to reduce sleeping in the daytime
▶ encourage the person to stay up later and not go to bed when it is still daylight
▶ assist with low-level activity, such as walking or listening to music, in the evening to divert restless evening behaviour
▶ encourage daily exercise
▶ perform relaxation techniques when the person is lying in bed
▶ play soft music
▶ chat with the person, provide reassurance and stay with them until they settle
▶ reduce the intake of stimulants, such as coffee, cola, tea, alcohol, chocolate and cigarette smoking, during the day and avoid after 5 pm
▶ offer a back rub or massage before bedtime
▶ avoid any tasks that upset the person or provide overstimulation in the afternoon and before bedtime.

Environmental factors

In addition to physical and psychological causes, environmental factors also compromise sleep (McCurry et al., 2006). Environmental factors are those relating to the immediate surroundings, including noise, temperature, lighting or changes to a familiar room, and can lead to disorientation or confusion (Martin et al., 2006). Others relate to the presence of family members, other patients or residents or the need for care by a professional carer or family member (Holland et al., 2008).

Strategies to deal with environmental factors that disrupt sleep

Strategies to address these environmental causes and minimise disruption to sleep are listed below. Carers should:
▶ avoid making changes to the room and maintain it in a familiar way to prevent confusion

- where practical, change the colour of the room to a restful colour, such as pink or lilac
- ensure the room is not too hot, cold, noisy or light
- supply comfortable night clothes
- keep the room dark during sleep, as shadows or light may wake the person or lead to hallucinations
- keep the room free of clutter and distractions
- create a home-like environment by using the person's own bed, bedcovers or comfortable pillow (if possible, place a favourite picture of a child or pet near the bed as this will promote a safe, comfortable feeling)
- use night lights to help the person see in the dark, this may also prevent confusion
- put clothing away so the person does not think they need to get up and dressed for the day
- if you are unable to get the person back to bed, try getting them to sleep in a recliner chair with the television on low volume.

Socio-cultural factors

Socio-cultural factors influence sleep habits and behaviour. Having an awareness of different cultural beliefs and practices and accommodating preferences for the person with dementia can assist in promoting sleep. Sleeping preferences to consider include:

- what time to sleep (e.g. a siesta in the daytime)
- where to sleep (e.g. in a bed, on a mat or on the floor)
- whether to sleep alone or to share a bed
- what nightclothes to wear
- what type of bed linen to use (e.g the number of pillows or blankets).

Communication considerations

If the person with dementia is waking at night, there are approaches you can use to enhance your communication with them. Generally, these are the same approaches you would use when communicating with a person with dementia at any time. If required, carers should try to:

- ▶ approach the person in a calm, slow manner, while talking softly
- ▶ stand still in front of the person and speak quietly – moving around is distracting
- ▶ touch the person's arm – this helps to keep their attention
- ▶ observe their non-verbal behaviour – this may give you some ideas about the problem
- ▶ be aware of your non-verbal language – the person with dementia will respond to the expression on your face and your stance
- ▶ remind the person it is night time
- ▶ point to the bed – this reinforces what you are saying
- ▶ use simple sentences to prevent confusion
- ▶ ask questions requiring only a yes or no answer
- ▶ avoid arguing with the person – if you are unable to resolve the situation, walk away and then come back later
- ▶ be patient
- ▶ always treat the person with sensitivity and respect.

Service referrals

There are services available to assist you in promoting sleep for the person with dementia. Services you can access easily for information and support include the:

- ▶ local doctor
- ▶ local community health centre
- ▶ Aged Care Information Line
- ▶ Commonwealth Carer Respite Centre
- ▶ National Dementia Helpline
- ▶ National Dementia Behaviour Management Advisory Service.

Conclusion

Sleep is an essential activity of living that maintains and restores mind and body health. Ageing and dementia can interfere with sleep and compromise the quantity and quality of sleep, impacting on the wellbeing of the person with dementia and you as their carer. Understanding that dementia is experienced differently amongst individuals and that there are many causes of sleep disturbance will assist you in determining the most appropriate strategies to use to promote sleep for the person with dementia. Communicating effectively and obtaining support from others when needed, such as family, friends or professional carers, will enhance the experience for you and the person with dementia.

References

Ancoli-Israel. S., & Vitiello, M. V. (2006). Sleep in Dementia [Editorial]. *The American Journal of Geriatric Psychiatry, 14*(2), 91–94.

Eeles, E. (2006). Sleep and its management in dementia. *Reviews in Clinical Gerontology, 16,* 59–70.

Gabelle, A., & Dauvilliers, Y. (2010). Sleep and dementia [Editorial]. *The Journal of Nutrition, Health and Aging, 14*(3), 201–202.

Harris, P., Nagy, S., & Vardaxis, N. (2009). *Mosby's Dictionary of Medicine, Nursing & Health Professions* (2nd ed.). Sydney: Mosby Elsevier.

Holland, K., Jenkins, J., Solomon, J., & Whittam, S. (Eds.). (2008). *Applying the Roper, Logan, Tierney model in practice* (2nd ed.). Sydney: Churchill Livingstone Elsevier.

Lee, D. R., & Thomas, A. J. (2011). Sleep in dementia and caregiving–assessment and treatment implications: A review. *International Psychogeriatrics, 23*(2), 190–201.

Lehne, R. (2010). *Pharmacology for nursing care* (7th ed.). St Louis, MO: Saunders Elsevier.

Marieb, E. (2012). *Essentials of human anatomy and physiology* (10th ed.). San Francisco: Benjamin Cummings.

Martin, J. L., Webber, A. P., Alam, T., Harker, J. O., Josephson, K. R., & Alessi, C. A. (2006). Daytime sleeping, sleep disturbance, and circadian rhythms in the nursing home. *The American Journal of Geriatric Psychiatry, 14*(2), 121–129.

McCurry, S. M., Vitiello, M. V., Gibbons, L. E., Logsdon, R. G., & Teri, L. (2006). Factors associated with caregiver reports of sleep disturbances in persons with dementia. *The American Journal of Geriatric Psychiatry, 14*(2), 112–120.

Porth, C. (2011). *Essentials of pathophysiology: Concepts of altered health states* (3rd ed.). Philadelphia: Lippincott Williams and Wilkins.

Waters, F., & Bucks, R. S. (2011). Neuropsychological effects of sleep loss: Implications for neuropsychologists. *Journal of the International Neuropsychological Society, 17,* 571–586.

Chapter 5

MANAGING CONTINENCE

Danielle McIntosh
HammondCare

Rebecca Forbes
HammondCare

Chapter outcomes

When you have completed this chapter you will be able to:

▶ understand what continence is and how issues can arise

▶ understand the impact that dementia can have on continence

▶ understand and implement effective strategies to promote independence in toileting.

Keywords

continence, emotional impact, assessment, routines, individualised care, environmental strategies

---

Introduction

Being able to use the toilet independently is a skill that is celebrated and praised in the early years of life with proclamations like 'You're a big boy/girl now!' Society places great importance on the hygienic management of bodily fluids and other by-products. It is therefore an emotional journey when a person starts to have problems managing these tasks and it is linked to a sense of shame and burden. It is estimated that 4.8 million Australians experience some form of bladder and bowel control issues (Continence Association of Australia, 2012). People have problems controlling their bladder and bowel for a variety of reasons, but for the purposes of this book we will focus on the reason being dementia. The strategies listed in this chapter are intended to help a person with dementia maintain their independence and dignity for longer. The main aim of effective care is to decrease distress for the person with dementia and their carer.

What is continence?

Continence is the ability to control the bladder (through urination) and the bowel (for faecal matter) (Hann et al., 2005). When someone has continence issues, it is referred to as 'incontinence'. This assumes that the person has total incapacity to be continent. In our experience, however, this is untrue. With the right support and a helpful environment, many people with dementia can be continent.

There are two types of continence issues: those caused by a medical problem (such as muscle weakness or disease) and those caused by what is termed 'functional incontinence'.

There are many medical and health reasons why someone may have issues with continence. Research shows that 1 in 3 women who give birth experience muscle weakness, frequently resulting in leakage of urine (National Continence Program, 2011). Other medical reasons include an atonic bladder (the inability of the bladder to stretch to hold normal volumes) and the inability of the bladder and bowel to empty properly. For more details, the Continence Foundation of Australia has a variety of easy-to-read resources (see <www.continence.org.au/>) or you can contact them on the National Continence Helpline (Ph: 1800 330066). Some types of dementia, such as dementia with Lewy Bodies and dementia secondary to Parkinson's disease, have a higher incidence of this type of incontinence (Idiaquez & Roman, 2011) due to deterioration in areas of the brain that control muscle impulses and movement. People with these types of dementia may also experience functional incontinence.

Functional incontinence refers to a situation when a person experiences incontinence, but muscle weakness or specific bladder or bowel diseases are not the cause. Often people with dementia will have this type of incontinence (Yap & Tan, 2006). Not being able to find the toilet in time or not recognising the urge to go to the toilet are common causes of functional incontinence. This chapter will focus on causes of functional incontinence and strategies to manage them.

How does having dementia impact on continence issues?

Based on our experiences caring for people with dementia, the following factors can create continence issues:

▶ The person may be unable to find the toilet or recognise what the toilet looks like (see Figure 5.1).

▶ The person may be unable to initiate, plan or perform the steps involved, or may get the order of the steps muddled (e.g. they might sit on the toilet seat before taking their pants down).

▶ The person may be unable to manipulate the buttons on their trousers or pull their skirt up to use the toilet. If in hospital, they might not know where to find the opening in the hospital gown.

▶ The person may not be physically able to walk or sit to use the toilet any more. The only option left is to use a bed pan, urinal or an incontinence aid. If they are not used to it, this may be an awful and confusing experience.

▶ The person may not recognise (or may misinterpret) the sensation of wanting to use the toilet. This could mean that when they do recognise the urge, they have too little time left and they can't hold on any more.

▶ Due to a short attention span, the person may not recognise that they are still urinating and may stand up before they have finished.

▶ The person may be stressed making it harder to concentrate or think. The emotional state of the person can negatively impact on continence issues. Feeling down decreases the attention you pay to your personal hygiene or needs. Some people can simply find going to the toilet very distressing. Stressful experiences include pain during urinating or bowel action, an inability to recognise the act of urinating/defecating or shame at having someone standing next to them in the bathroom.

▶ The person may be prescribed medications for other conditions, such as heart disease, and these may cause more frequent urination or have a laxative effect.

▶ If the person is having respite in residential care or is in hospital they may experience continence issues because:

　▷ the staff don't know their needs or routines

　▷ they don't know where the toilet is

　▷ their fluid intake is increased

　▷ they feel embarrassed or anxious about being accompanied when going to the toilet.

▶ The person may have a urinary tract infection, which can mean the passing of urine is painful or uncomfortable, resulting in a resistance to going to the toilet. Past experiences of pain might also affect the situation.

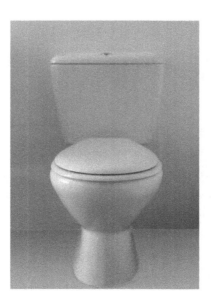

Source: Used with permission from HammondCare

Figure 5.1 All white toilet and tiles can cause difficulty for people with dementia

The impact of continence issues on the person and their carers

The impacts of the factors listed above include:

▶ **humiliation** of all involved due to embarrassing situations

▶ **constant worry** (about humiliation, especially if they have experienced it), which can lead to anxiety and depression

▶ **loss of independence**, self confidence and identity as an adult

▶ **dehydration**, which can occur if the amount the person drinks is restricted – this puts them at risk of developing a urinary tract infection and associated symptoms (such as confusion) and kidney disease

▶ **social isolation**, which can result from staying at home and not socialising with people to avoid the embarrassment of the person having an accident

▶ **carer stress and relationship breakdown**, which can result if the carer is not able to manage the continence of the person with dementia. They may feel there is no other option than placement in residential care. In these cases, carers may not be aware of useful strategies to implement (see the strategies section below).

Managing continence issues for the person with dementia

'Know the person' strategies

Better practice depends on an individualised approach and having strategies in place to suit the person is better than a 'one size fits all' approach. The following strategies will assist the carer in knowing what the person's toileting needs.

Know when the person goes to the toilet

Humans are creatures of habit. We tend to eat, drink and use the toilet at the same time every day. You may want to keep a 24-hour record with a diary or chart to help with this.

Find out what phrase the person uses to refer to going to the toilet

'I need to go to the toilet' is obvious, but some people might use a particular phrase or euphemism, such as 'spend a penny' or 'going to see a man about a dog'. This could be specific to their culture or first language.

Look out for non-verbal signs that the person needs to go the toilet

A person may not be able to say that they need to go to the toilet. However, they may display a non-verbal sign, such as squeezing their legs together, wringing their hands, furrowing their brow, looking agitated or breathing quickly but shallowly. This is often individual, so learn what to look out for.

Understand the person's cultural background

This will reduce problems and embarrassment. People from some cultural backgrounds may only be happy with help from a specific gender of staff.

Offer dignity and sensitivity

A person living with dementia is not incontinent deliberately. Toileting is a personal and private task and therefore we should offer as much privacy and dignity as possible. Objective and unemotional reassurance is better for the person.

Continence assessment strategies

Truly understanding the person's toileting needs and past experiences are important when developing strategies that work. To help assess a person's continence, some useful strategies and questions to ask are described below.

Note the amount

Are their pants or incontinence aid damp (indicating some leakage before using the toilet), wet (the person has urinated) or 'flooded' (indicating that they have urinated on a few occasions)? This indicates if the toilet is being used at all.

Note the frequency

How often and when does the person go to the toilet? Do they go before or after meals? Note if these tend to be the same every day – including the night is just as important (Kerr & Wilkinson, 2011).

Describe what happens

Describe what happens before, during and after the person has been incontinent. Were there events that could shed light on what happened? The quote below is an example:

> John was found outside, crying and with wet pants. When carers brought him back inside, they noticed that someone had put a sign near the toilet door warning them that the floor was slippery. John pointed to the sign and said 'out of order'.

Describe if the person has difficulty with other relevant tasks

If a person needs help with getting their pants on and doing up buttons in the morning, then it is likely that they will need help with these things throughout the day, including when going to the toilet.

Medical and medication review

Always investigate any underlying medical issues, such as urinary tract infections, to ensure that they are not the cause of continence issues. The general practitioner and local pharmacist can also review medications to determine if these could be contributing. Over-the-counter medications and vitamins and/or supplements could also have an impact.

Environmental strategies

Research has proved that an environment that provides cues and hints, rather than confuses and disables, benefits the person with dementia (Dementia Services Development Centre, 2011). Environmental strategies that might be useful are described below.

Locating the toilet

Have you ever needed to go to the toilet, but can't find it? Then, when you do find the toilets, the sign indicating the right door is confusing? This is what a person with dementia may experience all the time. To make the toilet as visible as possible (Namazi & Johnson, 1991):

▶ always keep the door to the toilet open
▶ place signs on the toilet door or in a hallway leading to the toilet
▶ use a picture of a toilet, rather than words
▶ keep a light on in the toilet, especially at night
▶ remove unnecessary clutter and equipment
▶ if possible, position the person's bed so that they can see the toilet from their bed.

Accessibility and ease

Make sure that the person is able to get on and off the toilet as independently and safely as possible. Raising the height of the seat and using grab rails can help. This equipment is readily available from chemists and hospitals. An occupational therapist can assist with the proper placement of these rails. Also remember to position the person as close to the toilet as possible. A bedside commode is an option if the toilet is too far away.

Colour contrast

The use of contrasting colour is helpful in assisting an older person with dementia to see objects more clearly. Use colour to highlight the:

▶ toilet door
▶ toilet seat (to define it from the rest of the toilet – see Figure 5.2)
▶ rails, toilet paper and toilet roll holder
▶ skirting (to define the floor and wall).

Lighting

Ways of lighting a room for someone with dementia include:

▶ increasing light levels to twice 'normal' levels, by opening curtains, adding more lights or increasing wattage

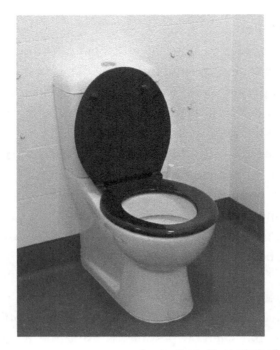

Source: Used with permission from HammondCare

Figure 5.2 Use colour contrast to help a person see the object

▶ using daylight whenever possible
▶ using lighting to highlight features in the bathroom – especially at night (McNair et al., 2011; also see Figure 5.3).

Set up the toilet and bathroom for the person

If the person is used to a certain layout in the toilet and/or bathroom, then it is important to maintain it. If they are used to a urinal or commode at night, then continue this. In winter, a heater can make sitting on the toilet more comfortable as the bathroom might be cold. An example is described below:

Tommy spent all day outside watching the sky, listening to the birds and working in the garden. He wasn't allowed inside unless he had taken off his garden clothes and had a wash. To save time and nagging, he used

a tree to relieve himself. When he moved into residential care, he sat outside all day and would use whatever he could find in the backyard for a toilet. Carers recognised his normal routine, so a tree was positioned in a discreet part of the garden. Tommy used the tree from then on.

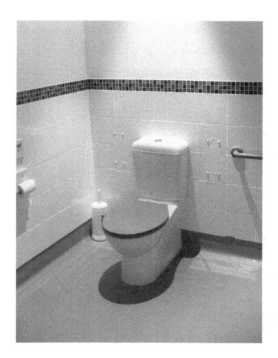

Source: Used with permission from HammondCare

Figure 5.3 Using lights can be effective in highlighting the toilet

Routines

Prompt the person

Prompt the person to go to the toilet at the times they usually go. Pay attention to any non-verbal signs and the physical environment, as something like the running water of a fountain can stimulate the bladder. Prompting may include verbally asking the person if they want to go to the toilet, showing them a picture of a toilet or pointing to the toilet when walking past it.

Assistance

It is important to know what assistance the person needs and will accept. Encourage as much independence as possible. If the person does not like receiving help, consider strategies of support without actually being near them (e.g. visual access to the toilet or verbal prompts rather than physical intervention). Ensure that the person's clothes aren't hindering them and consider how their clothes could be simplified (e.g. replacing trousers that have belts, buttons and zippers with elastic waisted trousers that are easy to pull down and up).

Positioning on the toilet

Ensure that the person is comfortable on the toilet and is sitting in a good position. Using a padded toilet seat may be helpful, especially if they are underweight. Some shorter people find a foot stool useful to bring their knees up higher than their hip, which is recommended for a full emptying of their bladder. However, people with dementia may find the footstool confusing and an obstacle, as it would not normally be associated with the toilet.

Encourage healthy practices

To encourage healthy practices for toileting, carers should:

▶ encourage the person with dementia to drink six to eight glasses of water a day
▶ encourage regular, but not overly frequent, toileting – the bladder needs to 'stretch' to hold an appropriate volume
▶ always ensure that the person's skin is cleaned and dried after each episode to promote good skin integrity
▶ choose the correct size and volume capacity incontinence aids for the person and situation – for example, a night aid holds greater volumes than a day aid (incontinence aids do not solve the issue of continence but when chosen and used correctly can provide dignity, comfort and confidence. Effective hygiene practice will also reduce the risk of urinary tract infection).

Conclusion

There are many continence-promoting strategies that can support a person with dementia. A well laid out environment can help a person to find and use the toilet. Incontinence aids with an established routine promote dignity. A person-centred approach based on knowing the person and understanding their needs is the key to continued quality of life.

References

Continence Association Australia. (2012). *About bladder and bowel health* [webpage]. Retrieved from http://www.continence.org.au/pages/about.html

Dementia Services Development Centre. (2011). *Dementia design audit tool.* Sydney: HammondPress. Available from http://www.dementiacentre.com.au

Hann, L., Keatley, C., O'Brien, B., & Schofield, A. (2005). *Help for people who care for someone with bladder and bowel problems.* Retrieved from http://www.bladderbowel.gov.au/assets/doc/ContinenceCarers.pdf

Idiaquez, J., & Roman, G. C. (2011). Autonomic dysfunction in neurodegenerative dementias. *Journal of the Neurological Sciences, 305*(1–2), 22–27.

Kerr, D., & Wilkinson, H. (2011). *Providing good care at night for older people: Practical approaches for use in nursing and care homes.* London: Jessica Kingsley Publishing. Available from http://www.dementiacentre.com.au

McNair, D. G., Cunningham, C., Pollock, R., & McGuire, B. (2011). *Light and lighting design for people with dementia.* Sydney: HammondPress. Available from http://www.dementiacentre.com.au

Namazi, K. H., & Johnson, B. D. (1991). Environmental effects on incontinence problems in Alzheimer's disease patients. *American Journal of Alzheimer's Disease and Other Dementias, 6*(6), 16–21.

National Continence Program. (2011).*One in three women who ever had a baby wet themselves!* Canberra: Commonwealth of Australia. Retrieved from http://www.bladderbowel.gov.au/assets/doc/OneInThree.pdf

Yap, P., & Tan, D. (2006). Urinary continence in dementia. *Australian Family Physician, 35*(4), 237–241.

Chapter 6

MANAGING CONSTIPATION

Danielle McIntosh
HammondCare

Rebecca Forbes
HammondCare

Chapter outcomes

When you have completed this chapter you will be able to:

▸ understand what constipation is and how it can be caused

▸ appreciate the impact that constipation can have on a person with dementia

▸ implement strategies that can be used to identify, manage and prevent constipation.

Keywords

constipation, causes, emotional impact, assessment, strategies

---

Introduction

Constipation is not a normal part of ageing (Kyle, 2011; World Gastroenterology Organisation, 2007) and should not be put up with (Brandt et al., 2005). It can be painful, frustrating and embarrassing. For a person with dementia it can also be frightening as they may not be able to understand why they are feeling unwell or may not be able to communicate what they are experiencing. This can prolong discomfort and hinder effective treatment.

What is constipation?

Constipation is not only the inability to open the bowels, but is also the infrequent passing of small or hard stools with or without straining (Bell et al., 2006; Better Health Channel, 2011). Between 15.3% and 30.7% of Australians experience constipation at some time (Peppas et al., 2008).

There are many causes of constipation. The most common are:

▶ not having enough fibre in your diet
▶ not drinking enough (especially water)
▶ holding on when you get an urge to open your bowels
▶ inactivity (especially not walking)
▶ taking certain medications (over-the-counter included) such as antidepressants, codeine, morphine and iron supplements
▶ incomplete emptying of the bowel
▶ having some form of urinary or faecal incontinence (Bolin et al., 2005; Continence Foundation of Australia, 2012; Hann et al., 2005).

How does having constipation impact people with dementia and their carers?

People with constipation might experience abdominal discomfort, pain, a lack of energy, a loss of appetite and/or emotional issues (Wald et al., 2007). People with dementia may also experience:

▶ a longer duration of side effects as they may not be able to communicate what is happening or how they are feeling
▶ feeling agitated and irritable, requiring additional reassurance
▶ a loss of independence, including a loss of dignity and self-worth
▶ an aversion to going out because of not feeling well or a fear of accidents such as overflow (uncontrollable bowel liquid) or diarrhoea (due to laxative use).

All of these symptoms may make the task of caring for the person with dementia more of a challenge for the carer. Sometimes a carer may take a person off their usual medication, commonly pain relief tablets, because it is causing or worsening their constipation. Remember, there are strategies that can be effective in managing constipation while maintaining other aspects of care, such as being pain free. Changes to medications are only one of many options.

If the person attends overnight or residential respite or is staying in hospital, they may eat unfamiliar foods, which may have an impact on their bowels. This may cause distress to the person with dementia and frustration for the carer, who may have put systems in place at home which are working, only to have them disrupted. Other factors that impact constipation include changes to the time of eating or the quantity of food. You should always inform the respite or hospital staff of specific bowel routines and foods eaten (or foods to be avoided).

Bill was very particular about what Rosemary ate, as she had a tendency to be constipated. When Rosemary went to respite for a week, Bill was not asked by the staff and he himself forgot to tell them what Rosemary has for breakfast. Rosemary helped herself to her favourite – cornflakes – every morning. She had not eaten them for so long! After three days, Rosemary had not opened her bowels. Bill became upset as he always gave Rosemary a high-fibre breakfast with prunes every morning as it helped keep her regular and comfortable.

How can constipation be managed for a person living with dementia?

There are many well-known strategies to help prevent constipation. While the science may not be strong to support them (Johanson & Kralstein, 2007), we have found that while some strategies may work well for some people, they don't for others. So, the key is to be aware of all the strategies and don't be afraid to try.

'Know the person' strategies

Treat the person with dignity and sensitivity

The person with dementia might not want to admit that they have a problem and might hide or ignore it. At other times, the person may not be able to remember when they last opened their bowels, so they will be oblivious to the issue. Being sensitive to their feelings will help you to avoid embarrassment for all involved.

Know the person's normal toileting routine

It is normal to open your bowels anywhere from daily to two or three times per week. As we tend to eat at the same time and eat the same types of food, we tend to open our bowels at similar times too. Knowing the person's normal routine will help you work out if the person has opened their bowels or not.

Know which words or language the person uses to refer to constipation

It is important to know how the person refers to going to the toilet. 'I can't go to the toilet' is fairly obvious, but some people might use a particular phrase or euphemism to say that they have been unable to open their bowels or that it hurts. These may include 'I can't do a number 2' or I'm unable to make a deposit'. Find out what phrase the person might use. They will understand what you are asking them and they might feel more comfortable with you using this. Also the question 'Have you opened your bowels today?' might be confusing if the person is not familiar with it.

Look for non-verbal signs that the person is experiencing constipation

Depending on the type of dementia or the length of time they have had dementia, a person may not be able to express verbally that they are constipated. Often, however, they will display a non-verbal sign, such as wringing their hands, scrunching their face, looking agitated or rubbing their stomach. They may also display more irritability, lethargy or lack of appetite.

Do they have a history of constipation?

If a person has a history of constipation, they are at risk of developing constipation again. Always ensure that this information is given to the person's general practitioner (GP), community service provider or residential care staff. It is better for the person if constipation can be prevented, rather than have them experience discomfort until it is resolved.

Constipation assessment and monitoring strategies

Having a thorough understanding of the person's bowel routine is important in trying to work out what strategies may be helpful. Sitting down and working through what the person experiences will help you plan the strategies you could use.

Be observant

Whilst it might seem gruesome, it is a good idea to be able to describe specific details about what the person is experiencing. When the person is on the toilet, discreetly watch or listen to see if the person is straining or showing any signs of pain or discomfort. If possible, try to have a look at what is in the toilet. The Bristol Stool Chart is a user-friendly scale that can help describe the type of stool. You can access a copy of the Bristol Stool chart from the Continence Foundation of Australia website <www.continence.org.au/pages/bristol-stool-chart.html>.

Monitor the opening of the person's bowels

Depending on the relationship with the person, and the person's ability to give an accurate answer, you could ask them outright or keep track of when they have opened their bowels. Keeping a simple diary can help carers keep track of what is happening over the week. If the person is not able to tell you accurately, you can look for evidence, such as any marks on the toilet bowl or even checking an incontinence aid (if worn).

What is their diet?

Are they eating enough fibre? Are they drinking enough? A diet high in fibre is recommended for the maintenance of a healthy bowel motion and in preventing constipation (Bolin et al., 2005). It is recommended that women eat 25 g of fibre per day and men 30 g per day.

Medical and medication review

Seek medical review

Speak with the person's GP regarding any ongoing constipation issues, as it is important to rule out any underlying medical conditions such as a bowel blockage or other health condition.

What medications is the person on?

Some medications can cause constipation as a possible side effect. Medications such as antidepressants, codeine-based pain relief drugs and iron supplements can increase the risk of constipation. Seek guidance from a pharmacist to identify if any of the medications they are taking might cause constipation. The person's GP may recommend medications that could help resolve and prevent further episodes of constipation. These include stool softeners and stimulants (e.g. laxatives).

Environmental strategies

All of the environmental strategies discussed in Chapter 5 on continence are relevant to constipation too. When the person needs to go to the toilet, it is important that they can find it and sit on it properly. Good dementia design is also good design for older people and people with disabilities. In fact, good dementia design is good design full stop.

Assistance

Know what assistance the person needs and will accept

As we discussed in the previous chapter on continence, supporting the person to do as much as they can is vital to maintain their dignity, self-worth and independence. Don't do everything for them, even though it might be tempting as it will save you time.

Positioning on the toilet

Ensure that the person is comfortable on the toilet and in a good sitting position. Some shorter people may find a footstool useful to bring their knees higher than their hips, which puts them in a good position for opening their bowels. However, people with dementia may find the footstool confusing (as it would not normally be associated with the toilet or bathroom). If used, you should also take care that it does not become an obstacle or a falls risk.

Encourage healthy practices

Encourage the person to drink six to eight glasses of water a day

As people get older they do not experience thirst as much and people with dementia may not be able to say that they are thirsty or help themselves to a drink. In the warmer months or even in winter, if there is heating on, the person may be at risk of dehydration. Having a jug of water with a glass on the kitchen bench or dining room table can be a good way to encourage the person to drink. You can also monitor how much they have drunk by checking the jug. Additionally, always serve drinks with meals. If a person does not like water, you can add cordial (diet or sugar-based) or fruit juice to the water to make it taste sweeter. Other sources of fluid can include milk, custard, jellies and iceblocks. An example of a different way of keeping the person with dementia hydrated is described below:

> Staff at a high-care facility noticed that residents did not like to drink much water, often pushing the glasses away or tipping them into the garden. Staff noticed, however, that the residents loved eating ice-cream. They decided to trial iceblocks every day in summer. The residents loved them as they said they were cool and reminded them of their childhood.

Ensure that the person is eating a balanced diet that is high in fibre

There are not many fruit juices that contain fibre, as most of it is removed in the juicing process. So whilst some people might swear by pear or prune juice, for example, you should take a cautious approach. Try it and see if it works. If it does not work, try other things. Some practical strategies to increase fibre intake include:

▶ adding 3 prunes to breakfast cereal (Attaluri et al., 2011)
▶ changing to a high-fibre breakfast cereal, such as wholegrain breakfast biscuits, porridge (Wisten & Messner, 2005) or other bran-based cereals
▶ eating wholemeal bread
▶ having a piece of fruit or a blended smoothie as a snack (fruit can be canned, fresh or cooked)
▶ having extra beans, corn, broccoli or carrots with your main meal.

Seek dietitian services

A dietitian can help if you are unsure of how to increase the amount of fibre in the person's diet and/or they have allergies or are on a pureed diet. The person's GP can refer you to a dietitian or you can contact the Dietitians Association of Australia <http://daa.asn.au/> for assistance and guidance in locating a dietitian. Most hospitals also have a nutrition and dietetics department.

Maintain skin integrity

If a person is constipated, they could experience small amounts of faecal incontinence, so always ensure that their skin is cleaned and dried after each episode.

Incontinence aids do not solve constipation

Incontinence aids do not solve constipation; however, they can help reduce the impact of overflow episodes on the person's skin and maintain the person's comfort and dignity.

There are other more intrusive procedures such as enemas and suppositories

While they have a place in the care of the person, especially when the constipation can't be resolved by other means, it is important to remember that more intrusive procedures can be frightening and quite unappealing to the person with dementia.

Conclusion

Despite a person having dementia, there are many strategies that can be put in place to maintain a healthy bowel routine and minimise the impact of constipation. These include:

▶ observing the person's body language and keeping a bowel diary/daily chart to help keep track and identify if they might be experiencing constipation

▶ having an environment that helps the person quickly and easily locate the toilet

▶ ensuring the person has a diet high in fibre and has six to eight glasses of water per day

▶ asking the person's GP or pharmacist if any medications they are taking could cause constipation. This can help by avoiding the problem before it starts to cause distress.

References

Attaluri, A., Donahoe, R., Valestin, J., & Rao, S. S. (2011). Randomised clinical trial: Dried plums (prunes) vs. psyllium for constipation. *Alimentary Pharmacology and therapeutics 33(7),* 822–828.

Bell, J., Bolin, T., Cowen, A., Gullotta, J., Georgeou, G., Kellow, J., Korman, M., & Nicholson, F. (2006). *Constipation and bloating.* Randwick, NSW: The Gut Foundation. Retrieved from http://www.gutfoundation.com/publications-1/constipation-and-bloating-2006

Better Health Channel. (2011). *Fact sheet: Constipation.* Retrieved from http://www.betterhealth.vic.gov.au/bhcv2/bhcpdf.nsf/ByPDF/Constipation/$File/Constipation.pdf

Bolin, T., Cowen, A., Korman, M., & Stanton, R. (2005). *Dietary fibre and health.* Randwick, NSW: The Gut Foundation. Retrieved from http://www.gutfoundation.com/publications-1/dietary-fibre-and-health-2002

Brandt, L. J., Prather, C. M., Quigley, E. M., Schiller, L.R., Schoenfeld, P., & Talley, N. J. (2005). Systematic review on the management of chronic constipation in North America. *The American Journal of Gastroenterology 100,* Suppl 1, s5–s21.

Continence Foundation of Australia. (2012). *Constipation* [webpage]. Retrieved from http://www.continence.org.au/pages/constipation.html

Hann, L., Keatley, C., O'Brien, B., & Schofield, A. (2005). *Help for people who care for someone with bladder and bowel problems.* Retrieved from http://www.bladderbowel.gov.au/assets/doc/ContinenceCarers.pdf

Johanson, J. F., & Kralstein, J. (2007). Chronic constipation: A survey of the patient perspective. *Alimentary Pharmacology and Therapeutics, 25*(5), 599–608.

Kyle, G. (2011). Managing chronic constipation. *Journal of Community Nursing, 25*(5), 4–9.

Peppas, G., Alexiou, V. G., Mourtzoukou, E., & Falagas, M. E. (2008). Epidemiology of constipation in Europe and Oceania: A systematic review. *BMC Gastroenterology, 8*(1), 5. Retrieved from http://www.biomedcentral.com/1471-230X/8/5

Wald, A., Scarpignato, C., Kamm, M. A., Mueller-Lissner, S., Helfrich, I., Schuijt, C., Bubeck, J., Limoni, C., & Petrini, O. (2007). The burden of constipation on quality of life: Results of a multinational survey. *Alimentary Pharmacology and Therapeutics, 26*(2), 227–236.

Wisten, A., & Messner, T. (2005). Fruit and fibre (Pajala porridge) in the prevention of constipation. *Scandinavian Journal of Caring Sciences, 19*(1), 71–76.

World Gastroenterology Organisation. (2007). *Practice guidelines: Constipation.* Retrieved from http://www.worldgastroenterology.org/assets/downloads/en/pdf/guidelines/05_constipation.pdf

Chapter 7

BEHAVIOURAL CHALLENGES

Daniel Nicholls
University of Canberra

Chapter outcomes

When you have completed this chapter you will be able to:

▸ recognise behaviours that are concerning and challenging

▸ recognise feelings and responses that are evoked in the carer

▸ build strategies for concerns and challenges.

Keywords

behaviours, challenges, wandering, carer feelings, strategies

---

Introduction

In this chapter, how to manage behaviours that can be quite distressing for both the person with dementia and carers will be discussed. These behaviours are labelled concerning and challenging because they require carers to confront their own feelings and patience (Cubit et al., 2007). This chapter will look at the behaviours themselves, the feelings they evoke in carers and ways of dealing with both the behaviours and those feelings. The goal is to provide strategies that will lead to the best possible outcomes for carers and the person experiencing dementia.

What are challenging behaviours?

Generally, we think about aggression as the behaviour that causes carers the most concern and that presents the greatest challenge (Moyle et al., 2011). Aggression is when someone is verbally abusive or physically acts out, hitting, scratching or biting. It is a behaviour often linked to anger (Lochman et al., 2010). The difference between anger and aggression, however, is that anger is an emotion while aggression is an action directed at someone. Someone can be angry without being aggressive and aggression often can have nothing to do with anger. In some cases, and especially in people with dementia, aggression may result from frustration or fear (Bidewell & Chang, 2011). Imagine that you are trying to do up your shirt buttons, your hands are shaking and someone is telling you to hurry up. You can become so frustrated that you lash out. Or imagine that you feel trapped behind a door that you can't open; not knowing where you are or why you are there, then someone you don't recognise takes you by the arm. Your sudden fear can cause you to lash out. The question that will be asked in this chapter is 'What is the real challenge for us? The behaviour or the feelings behind it of anger, frustration or fear or a combination of these?'

Other behaviours that carers may find concerning and challenging include isolation, interference, wandering, screaming, the inability to sleep, food and fluid refusal (Chang & Roberts, 2011), and refusal to be assisted. The first five of these behaviours are to do with influences occurring within the person that may have effects on others. For example, isolation may be an expression of inability or an unwillingness to connect socially for any number of reasons, including depression or dislike of groups, open spaces or noisy environments. Interference certainly affects others and can lead to violent verbal or physical exchanges. The same could be said of screaming, which can be attributed to neurological factors or can be a learned behaviour. Wandering is a common problem and will be discussed below. The inability to sleep is well addressed by Bloom et al. (2009) and is talked about more specifically in Chapter 4. The final two refusal behaviours are to do with resistance to the will of others. This resistance, however, is usually not the wilful resistance to external controls often associated with ageing (Powell, 2009), but may be attributed to misinterpretation of another's intentions. Sometimes resistance can also be related to depression (Durand et al., 2009).

Feelings and responses evoked in the carer

It is clear that the challenging behaviours of those with dementia have effects on other people, namely the carer. Aggression from the person with dementia may lead to feelings of fear or anger in the carer, interference may lead to feelings of frustration and resistance may lead to feelings of annoyance. Behaviours and feelings also occur in a broader context. For example, as I am trying to assist the person with dementia with their clothing I am also aware that I have other pressing obligations. The feelings that occur in the carer can be transferred back to the person with dementia, intended or not. In other words, both the person and the carer may be locked in a 'battle of wills'. The difference is that the person with dementia is not able to 'will' something in the same way as the carer. The person with advanced dementia reacts to immediate stimuli and is not able to make longer term goals or plans, thus affecting the way they engage with other people (Yarry, Judge & Orsulic-Jeras, 2010). The immediate goal for a person with dementia may be to 'see what happens next'. To a carer this may appear like a form of passivity and thus evoke feelings of frustration in the carer. An understanding carer, however, will know that there is no intention to frustrate. Knowing this will free the carer from unnecessary and distressing feelings that may lead to abrupt and careless actions. However, it takes some work to acquire this knowledge and to be able to regulate feelings in the caring role. Acquiring this knowledge and regulating feelings are key parts of any behaviour management strategy.

How do we deal with our own feelings?

Knowledge itself can assist carers to feel more relaxed in the caring role. Once the carer sees that the person has no intention to hurt or frustrate, they can immediately obtain some distance from the situation. Also, once the carer sees that their own actions and words can produce negative effects in the person they can guard against inflaming a situation through actions and words of their own. For example, words carers use may seem harsh and critical to the person and may trigger responses linked to the person's past, of which the person has no conscious recollection.

Knowledge, however, is not sufficient. Feelings will continue to emerge in the carer despite their knowledge and best intentions, for carers also bring to the relationship their own buried memories. As you reflect on your feelings it is not necessary to dredge up those memories, but it is necessary to deal with the feelings. Thus, it is important to design a personal strategy before you attempt to design strategies to deal with the behaviour(s) (Nicholls, Anderson & Cross, 2011).

Personal strategies for dealing with carer concern

Recognise that the feelings are there

As a carer, if you don't recognise your own feelings you may act in ways that you wouldn't normally consider acceptable. For example, if you don't recognise your feelings of frustration you may act in an abrupt and dismissive way towards the person with dementia or someone else. Later, you may be annoyed with yourself for the way that you acted, not recognising that your own behaviour was a result of your frustration. In recognising feelings you also need to accept them. This means that you don't blame yourself for having the feelings. It is important to merely notice your feelings and to sit with them for a while.

Reorganise your schedule to find time to reflect

If you are constantly 'on the go', never resting, it will be difficult for you to find time to notice your feelings. Try to find the time to sit quietly by yourself to allow yourself to notice your feelings. You can do this in stages. Sometimes all it takes is a five-minute 'breather', to allow your body and mind to relax sufficiently so you can notice your feelings. This can be followed by a longer time when you completely rest your body and mind.

Rest when you can to stop and think

Resting is very important to allow carers to get some perspective on things. Make sure you find a quiet space and make yourself comfortable. It can be in a corner of the garden or at the kitchen table. Some people go for a long walk where all their usual distractions are far away. So resting doesn't necessarily mean sitting still. The important thing is that you find a space to stop and think. What is stopped is your usual activity.

Reflect on your feelings

This means that you look inwards at the feelings and see them for what they are. You may be feeling angry, but when you reflect on this anger you may find that it is related to lack of information or a lack of certainty. In this way, you start to see that you may need more information about a particular matter. Recognising this need can immediately diffuse your anger as you start to think of ways of getting the information you need. Other feelings you may need to reflect on are sadness, annoyance, guilt, jealousy and even happiness and joy. There are obviously more feelings than these and feelings will not be the same for any two people. Reflection on feelings can also be done with a colleague or friend. Find time to sit down with someone to talk things over.

Re-establish internal harmony and control

Control here means a feeling of safety and security. If feelings are allowed free rein they can have unwanted effects. For example, uncontrolled anger can lead to aggression as was discussed previously. Similarly, uncontrolled guilt can lead to self-loathing and uncontrolled joy can lead to embarrassing interactions. In establishing your own internal harmony you are in a better position to assist the person with dementia to have a safe and secure environment, both internally and externally.

Remind yourself of where you are and why you are here

Establishing this internal harmony and control is essential for you to deal with the situation you are in with the person with dementia. Remind yourself of your responsibility for this particular person who has difficulty in caring for her or himself.

Strategies for dealing with challenging behaviours

Don't engage in the same way

Engagement is the way that people connect with others. It refers to a person's verbal and non-verbal interactions. Try something different if what you have been saying, acting or doing isn't working. This doesn't mean being inconsistent with behaviour management. It means looking at the way you are engaging the person in that behaviour management and seeing if you can act differently. For example, you might smile brightly rather than looking worried and busy. This may relax the person who otherwise might take on and mimic your worried and busy look. You can also stop what you are saying or doing to distract the person from a focus that is causing them distress.

Develop a way of standing back to survey the situation

This can happen after the event so that you can develop strategies for the future or it can happen at the time of a concerning situation so that you can better manage it as it is occurring. You can stop and have a look around to see what's happening. In both cases, you need to carefully examine the immediate environment. For example, is there something in the environment that is upsetting the person? Is there a sheet caught around the person's leg? By standing back you will find many instances like this. The light may be too bright, there may be an unpleasant smell or the person's pyjamas may be wet and uncomfortable.

Try distraction from the current activity to something else

Sometimes a person with dementia may become fixated on a particular object or activity. You may find it difficult to engage with them or to assist them to move on to another activity. If you concentrate your efforts on moving them from what they are doing to something else you may find that they become even more resistant. In order to re-direct their attention you need to re-direct your own attention. For example, when the person is fixated on trying to open a locked door you can say something like 'I like your new dress. It's very beautiful. Are the flowers in the pattern roses or tulips?' This kind of statement will take the person's attention away from the activity that is frustrating them. Similarly, if someone is continually wandering you can assist them by finding another activity that will engage their attention.

Do something different

Similar to distraction, this is about activity that redirects the attention and focus of the person. Someone who is isolated and withdrawn can be activated with the introduction of a new activity. It might be an activity such as going for a walk in a new direction, baking a cake together, arranging flowers in a vase or trying on some new clothes. It can even be an activity that only lasts for the time that the person is able to keep their intention focussed (MacPherson et al., 2009). This area is further explored in Chapter 11 on mental stimulation.

Do something that will provide immediate comfort and pleasure

Immediate comfort and pleasure can be provided in many simple ways such as a soft touch to the face, fresh pyjamas, a pillow, a warm blanket or a pleasant word in a friendly voice. Other examples of comfort and pleasure that we sometimes overlook for those we care for include warm water to wash hands, the smell of fresh flowers, a cool breeze on a hot summer's day, a warm drink at night or a cool drink during the day. We sometimes forget the simple basics of comfort that can provide immediate pleasure and evoke a happy response.

Wandering: a particular challenge

Wandering may be caused by many factors that are often difficult to pinpoint (Better Health Channel, 2012). The person may be responding to an internal dialogue or have a sudden urge to return to a former residence. It is not difficult to imagine a confused state where external stimuli both combine and conflict with internal perceptions and anxieties. For example, the environment may be misinterpreted as hostile or a particular person may be perceived as an aggressor. Try to think about what this might be like for the person with dementia; it can be quite frightening. In keeping with the emphasis on providing safety and security for a person with dementia you must do everything in your power to minimise the risk of the person suddenly becoming frightened or experiencing a need to wander away.

There are many well-known strategies for ensuring that the environment is safe and secure. For example, the use or non-use of contrasting colours to show the person where they are located or to distract them from going where they shouldn't go. Having adequate and attractive places where the person can exercise in safety is also important (Kelly, Innes & Dincarlsan, 2011). The environment must not be prison-like as that may encourage the person to want to 'escape'. There are many other simple strategies that you must constantly remember to revise. For example, in case the person with dementia goes missing, ensuring that there is a recent, good quality photo of the person on file, that identification and contact phone numbers are located on the person and ensuring that neighbours are aware of the person's dementia. Community support is the best protection for both the person with dementia and those who care for them. Write your own list of strategies, including emergency contact phone numbers, and keep it in a place where you can refer to it whenever you need to. You also need to remember that the person with dementia may have no awareness that they had wandered away, therefore it is pointless to act negatively towards them when they return. A negative and critical attitude may exacerbate the situation; always remain calm, pleasant and matter-of-fact.

Conclusion

The chapter has presented some very simple strategies in assisting carers and the person with dementia to deal with behaviours that may be distressing for both. In practising these strategies carers come to realise that, depending on the severity of the dementia, the person is very often unable to exercise internal controls over their behaviour. The control lies with you, the carer, and supporters of the person with dementia. Since the control lies with you it is important that you look at yourself, your own attitudes and behaviours. It is also important that you look after yourself so that you can remain centred and objective. When you become practised with these strategies you will start to reframe the behaviours as no longer concerning or challenging, but rather as part of the interesting and changing fabric of the person's life. You will become more relaxed and thus better able to provide a safe and pleasant environment for both the person with dementia and yourself.

References

Better Health Channel (BHC). (2012). *Fact sheet: Dementia and wandering.* Retrieved from http://www.betterhealth.vic.gov.au/bhcv2/bhcpdf.nsf/ByPDF/Dementia_and_wandering/$File/Dementia_and_wandering.pdf

Bidewell, J., & Chang, E. (2011). Managing dementia agitation in residential aged care. *Dementia, 10*(3), 299–315.

Bloom, H. G., Ahmed, I., Alessi, C. A., Ancoli-Israel, S., Buysse, D. J., Kryger, M. H., Phillips, B. A., Thorpy, M. J., Vitiello, M. V., & Zee, P. C. (2009). Evidence-based recommendations for the assessment and management of sleep disorders in older persons. *Journal of the American Geriatrics Society, 57*(5), 761–789.

Chang, C., & Roberts, B. (2011). Strategies for feeding patients with dementia. *American Journal of Nursing, 111*(4), 36–44.

Cubit, K., Farrell, G., Robinson, A., & Myhill, M. (2007). A survey of the frequency and impact of behaviours of concern in dementia on residential aged care staff. *Australasian Journal on Ageing, 26*(2), 64–70.

Durand, M., James, A., Ravishankar, A., Bamrah, A. S., & Purandare, N. B. (2009). Domiciliary and day care services: Why do people with dementia refuse? *Aging & Mental Health, 13*(3), 414–419.

Kelly, F., Innes, A., & Dincarslan, O. (2011). Improving care home design for people with dementia. *Journal of Care Services Management, 5*(3), 147–155.

Lochman, J. E., Barry, T., Powell, N., & Young, L. (2010). Anger and aggression. In D. W. Nangle, D. J. Hansen, C. A. Erdley, & P. J. Norton (Eds.), *Practitioner's Guide to Empirically Based Measures of Social Skills* (pp. 155–166). New York: Springer.

MacPherson, S., Bird, M., Anderson, K., Davis, T., & Blair, A. (2009). An art gallery access programme for people with dementia: 'You do it for the moment'. *Aging & Mental Health, 13*(5), 744–752.

Moyle, W., Murfield, J. E., Griffiths, S. G., & Venturato, L. (2011). Care staff attitudes and experiences of working with older people with dementia. *Australasian Journal on Ageing, 30*(4), 186–190.

Nicholls, D., Anderson, B., & Cross W. (2011). Nurses health and self care in nursing. In K. Edward, I. Munro, A. Robins, & A. Welch (Eds.), *Mental health nursing: Dimensions of praxis* (pp. 483–502). London: Oxford University Press.

Powell, J. L. (2009). Social theory, aging, and health and welfare professionals: A Foucauldian 'toolkit'. *Journal of Applied Gerontology, 28*(6), 669–682.

Yarry, S. J., Judge, K. S., & Orsulic-Jeras, S. (2010). Applying a strength-based intervention for dyads with mild to moderate memory loss: Two case examples. *Dementia, 9*(4), 549–557.

Chapter 8

PAIN

Sara Karacsony
South Western Sydney Local Health District

Michel Edenborough
University of Western Sydney

Chapter outcomes

When you have completed this chapter you will be able to:

▸ identify possible causes of pain

▸ recognise behaviours that may be a sign of pain

▸ help make the person with dementia more comfortable and manage their pain.

Keywords

behaviour, assessment, management, analgesia, comfort care

Introduction

Pain can be a common problem for many people throughout the course of their dementia because, although dementia does not usually cause pain in itself, older people with dementia often have one or more painful conditions.

What does pain mean?

My whole body is sore. It hurts to move and it hurts to sit. A man has come to see me and tells me that I have arthritis. I laugh at him and

tell him: 'At my age? You must be joking!' He tells me I'm 86 and it's
common at my age and [he] will give me some medicine. I spit in his
face because he's lying (Regnard & Huntley, 2006, p. 25).

Pain is an unpleasant and very individual experience for anybody. For this reason, a person's own explanation of pain is the most reliable and carers need to believe what the person says. For people who have dementia and who may no longer be able to tell you about their pain, carers need to consider non-verbal cues and behavioural observation when assessing for pain (Eritz & Hadjistavropoulos, 2011; Kaasalainen, 2007).

Pain is not a normal part of the ageing process, although persistent pain increases with age and illness (Australian Pain Society, 2005). Many older people, with or without dementia, may adopt a long-suffering attitude and accept pain as part of becoming 'old'. A concern about taking strong medications and their side effects, a reluctance to complain and doubts about the effectiveness of pain relief all hinder effective pain assessment (McAuliffe et al., 2009).

Despite the misconception, even among health professionals, people with dementia *do* experience pain because the parts of the brain that interpret pain messages remains intact even though the processing and perception of pain may be altered (Gallagher & Long, 2011). In fact, people with dementia may experience more pain than other people with painful conditions because their pain is often under-recognised and under-treated (Eritz & Hadjistavropoulos, 2011; Federico, 2009; Gallagher & Long, 2011; McAuliffe et al., 2009). This is because people with dementia are less able to express their experience of pain, which may be the reason for behavioural responses, such as resisting care. Research has found that chronic pain, in particular, is under-recognised and under-treated in aged care residents, even in those residents with early stage dementia who were still able to say they had pain (McAuliffe et al., 2009). It is estimated up to 83% of patients with dementia experience pain at some point, with pain increasing as the dementia progresses to the end stage and death (Van der Steen, 2010).

Recognising signs of pain

Pain impacts on a person's activities, wellbeing and enjoyment of daily life and can contribute to or worsen physical and psychological problems. There is a link between pain and behavioural and psychiatric symptoms such as socially inappropriate behaviour, resisting care, abnormal thought processes and delusions (Tosato et al., 2011). Signs of unrelieved pain may include agitation and restlessness, aggression, uncooperativeness, wandering and pacing, yelling, calling out and screaming. Insomnia, loss of appetite and undernutrition, depression and further cognitive and functional decline may also develop (Federico, 2009; Gallagher & Long, 2011; Rabins, Lyketsos & Steele, 2006).

Challenging behaviours can have a significant effect on caregivers, so it is important for carers to be able to recognise and interpret behaviours that may be a sign of pain. The detection of pain is the first step in the process of pain assessment. As a carer, the second step is to discuss with the person's general practitioner (GP) or community nurse (or inform the registered nurse) that you suspect pain, which can then lead to effective treatment with analgesia, other non-medication strategies and complementary therapies.

What are some possible causes of pain?

You may already know what is causing pain; however, possible causes of pain to be aware of include sore gums, broken teeth and cavities, headaches, back pain, osteoarthritis, hip fractures, constipation, burning on urination, pressure ulcers, skin rashes, sore throats and colds (Rabins et al., 2006). The experience of pain can vary according to whether the type of pain is chronic or acute.

What are the different types of pain?

Chronic pain

Pain from pre-existing conditions such as arthritis, musculoskeletal problems, osteoporosis, degenerative disc disease, hip pain, back pain, ulcers and complications of diabetes or cancer is also described as chronic pain. This pain is often ongoing, lasting longer than three to six months. Chronic pain can be more difficult to recognise in individuals who cannot communicate, as the normal signs that accompany acute pain, such as a fast heart or pulse rate, guarding or holding a part of the body and pallor, are absent. It may also be difficult to pinpoint exactly where the pain is and there may be no behavioural reactions until the person moves. An obvious tenderness when the person is being touched may indicate chronic pain (Gibson, Scherer & Goucke, 2004).

Acute pain

Acute pain usually comes on suddenly, is severe and can cause sweating, a fast heart and pulse rate and nausea. It may result in the person crying or yelling, grimacing, rubbing or protecting the affected area (Gibson et al., 2004). This type of pain can be associated with angina, urinary tract infections, urinary retention, constipation, chest infections, headaches or other injuries such as a skin tear or bruising.

Incident pain

Incident pain results from a specific event or activity such as having a wound dressed or being transferred from bed to chair. Incident pain can be prevented or minimised by giving analgesia before the event that causes the pain (Australian Department of Health and Ageing, 2006).

What are the different causes of pain?

Within the three types of pain described above, pain is further categorised into three groups:

▶ nociceptive pain (tissue pain) – examples are cellulitis of the leg, pressure ulcers, bowel obstructions or cancer metastases
▶ neuropathic pain (nerve pain) – examples include sciatica pain or pain triggered by movement or touch
▶ pain related to psychological or psychiatric factors (Australian Pain Society, 2005).

Pain threshold

Each person's pain threshold is different. A person's perception of pain is influenced by their past pain experiences, as well as social, physical and environment factors. These factors affect a person's ability to manage or tolerate their pain. Table 8.1 lists the common factors that influence a person's pain threshold.

Table 8.1 Factors in the threshold of pain

Threshold lowered	Threshold raised
▸ Insomnia	▸ Relief of other symptoms
▸ Fatigue	▸ Sleep
▸ Anxiety	▸ Sympathy
▸ Fear	▸ Understanding
▸ Anger	▸ Relaxation
▸ Depression	▸ Reduction in anxiety
▸ Mental isolation	▸ Analgesia

Source: Palliative Care Australia, 2006, p. 9

What behaviours indicate pain?

Any new behaviour or sign may indicate pain and carers need to observe the person carefully to see whether, for example, the person is limping, resisting care or becoming tense and distressed. A good way to start identifying the cause of pain begins with asking. Genuine concern and carefully worded questions, allowing time for responses, will help. Questions include 'Are you in pain?', 'Does it hurt anywhere?' and 'Do you have any aching or soreness?' (Australian Pain Society, 2005, p. 2). For people who are unable to understand or tell you the location of pain, carefully observing what the person is doing may provide clues as to the level of their pain and what may be causing it. Table 8.2, on the following page, outlines some of the common pain–related behaviours.

Table 8.2 Common pain behaviours in cognitively impaired elderly persons

Characteristic	Behaviour
Facial expressions	▸ Slight frown, sad or frightened face ▸ Grimacing, wrinkled forehead, closed or tightened eyes ▸ Any distorted expression ▸ Rapid blinking
Verbalisations, vocalisations	▸ Sighing, moaning or groaning ▸ Grunting, chanting or calling out ▸ Noisy breathing ▸ Asking for help ▸ Verbally abusive
Body movements	▸ Rigid, tense body posture or guarding ▸ Fidgeting ▸ Increased pacing or rocking ▸ Restricted movement ▸ Gait or mobility changes
Changes in interpersonal interactions	▸ Aggressive, combative or resisting care ▸ Decreased social interactions ▸ Socially inappropriate or disruptive ▸ Withdrawn
Changes in activity patterns or routines	▸ Refusing food or appetite change ▸ Increase in rest periods ▸ Sleep or rest pattern changes ▸ Sudden cessation of common routines ▸ Increased wandering
Mental status changes	▸ Crying or tears ▸ Increased confusion ▸ Irritability or distress

Note: Some patients demonstrate little or no specific behaviour associated with severe pain.

Source: Used with permission from the American Geriatrics Society, 2002, p. S211

How to assess pain

Even in severe dementia, an assessment of pain is possible. A GP can perform a thorough physical examination along with obtaining a general medical history from you, including the person's pain history. This information will assist in the prognosis, as well as identifying which treatments and medications will be of benefit.

As carers, you know the person best; their regular habits and characteristics, likes and dislikes, and you probably have an intuitive sense of what the pain may be. This familiarity and an individual approach is helpful for all carers in interpreting and evaluating changes in the person's behaviour (McAuliffe et al., 2009) and deciding whether it should be communicated to their GP.

Being involved in the process of assessment and management is important to ensure the best outcomes are achieved for the person and that their wishes for treatment options and overall care are taken into consideration if medical procedures are necessary (Australian Pain Society, 2005).

Pain assessment

Pain in people with dementia is assessed using a number of key indicators. These include:

▶ whether pain is present
▶ how intense the pain is
▶ where the pain is located
▶ what is causing the pain.

Consideration needs to be given to the person with dementia's pain history and any relevant factors that may affect reporting pain or the amount and type of pain potentially being experienced. Regnard and Huntley (2006) suggest pain stems from emotional, physical or psychological distress. Therefore, as carers, knowing the individual and having rapport is valuable in recognising their particular communication of pain.

How to manage pain

Shega et al. (2006) examined pain management and the use of over-the-counter and prescribed medications amongst people with dementia and found that two-thirds of people in their study were experiencing pain and not using analgesics. In addition, those who were taking an analgesic were unlikely to be prescribed an opioid, such as morphine, which can be used to manage moderate to severe pain. Treating pain promptly by using analgesics and other therapies on a regular basis is important for effective pain management. It is also important to discuss pain management with their GP. Older people tend to be more sensitive to medicine and therefore require assessment to evaluate their comfort level and effectiveness of the medication.

What other strategies relieve pain?

Carers may consider other pain management strategies, focusing on the individual, their likes and dislikes, preferences and wishes. Simple strategies to promote comfort include repositioning, verbal reassurance and a supportive presence. High-touch strategies are non-invasive comfort measures designed to provide comfort, relieve discomfort and physical pain. Also see Chapter 10 on complementary therapies.

These alternative strategies include:

▶ massage therapy, which may relieve pain and discomfort of muscles and joints

▶ aromatherapy and the use of essential oils, such as lavender, geranium and marjoram, which may have a calming effect and add to a sense of comfort

▶ tranquil music and nature sounds, which may assist in promoting relaxation and decreasing anxiety

▶ the use of warmth and coolness on the body. Warmth has been found to stimulate the production of the body's own chemical opioids, so the application of a warm towel or wheat pack can be comforting. As well, a cold or cool towel can suppress the release of products from tissue damage (Australian Department of Health and Ageing, 2006).

Conclusion

Pain in people with dementia is under-recognised and under-treated. We know pain impacts on a person's quality of life and sense of wellbeing, leading to a decline in function, physical and psychological problems. Challenging behaviours, such as agitation, may be the result of pain and should prompt carers to carefully assess for possible pain. Recognising, interpreting and responding to the needs of older people with dementia, especially those who are unable to communicate in words, is the first step in treating pain. It is important to use analgesics on a regular basis and continue to assess the comfort level of the person with dementia to see if this is working. Verbal reassurance, playing music that a person enjoys or a gentle hand or foot massage can all bring comfort, as well as help carers feel they are doing something to help relieve pain.

References

American Geriatrics Society. (2002). The management of persistent pain in older persons: AGS panel on persistent pain in older persons. *Journal of the American Geriatrics Society, Clinical Practice Guidelines, 50*, Supplement 6, s205–s224.

Australian Department of Health and Ageing. (2006). *Guidelines for a palliative approach in residential aged care.* Canberra: Australian Department of Health and Ageing.

Australian Pain Society. (2005). *Pain in residential aged care facilities. Management strategies.* North Sydney, NSW: Australian Pain Society.

Eritz, H., & Hadjistavropoulos, T. (2011). Do informal caregivers consider nonverbal behavior when they assess pain in people with severe dementia? *Journal of Pain, 12*(3), 331–339.

Federico, A. (2009). Assessing pain in patients with dementia. *Nursing, 39*(12), 64.

Gallagher, M., & Long, C. O. (2011). Advanced dementia care: Demystifying behaviors, addressing pain, and maximizing comfort. *Journal of Hospice and Palliative Nursing, 13*(2), 70–78.

Gibson, S., Scherer, S., & Goucke, R. (2004). *Guidelines for residential care. Stage 1: Preliminary field-testing and preparations for implementation. Final report.* Perth: Australian Pain Society and the Australian Pain Relief Association Pain Management.

Kaasalainen, S. (2007). Assessment. Pain assessment in older adults with dementia: Using behavioral observation methods in clinical practice. *Journal of Gerontological Nursing, 33*(6), 6–10.

McAuliffe, L., Nay, R., O'Donnell, M., & Fetherstonhaugh, D. (2009). Pain assessment in older people with dementia: Literature review. *Journal of Advanced Nursing, 65*(1), 2–10.

Palliative Care Australia. (2006). *Guidelines for a palliative approach in residential aged care: Pain assessment and management.* Retrieved from http://www.agedcare.pallcare.org.au/LinkClick.aspx?fileticket=zSiFoEoP5CE%3d&tabid=828&mid=1381

Shega, J. W., Hougham, G. W., Stocking, C. B., Cox-Hayley, D., & Sachs, G. A. (2006). Management of noncancer pain in community-dwelling persons with dementia. *Journal of American Geriatric Society, 54*, 1892–1897.

Rabins, P. V., Lyketsos, C. G., & Steele, C. D. (2006). *Practical dementia care* (2nd ed.). New York: Oxford University Press.

Regnard, C., & Huntley, M. (2006). Managing the physical symptoms of dying. In J. C. Hughes (Ed.), *Palliative care in severe dementia.* London: MA HealthCare Limited.

Tosato, M., Lukas, A., van der Roest, H., Danese, P., Antocicco, M., Finne-Soveri, H., & Onder, G. (2011). Association of pain with behavioral and psychiatric symptoms among nursing home residents with cognitive impairment: Results from the SHELTER study. *Pain, 153*(2), 305–310.

Van der Steen, J. (2010). Dying with dementia: What we know after more than a decade of research. *Journal of Alzheimer's Disease, 22*(1), 37–55.

Chapter 9

MEDICATIONS

Kaniez Baig
bioCSL

Chapter outcomes

When you have completed this chapter you will be able to:

▶ understand how medications assist in the treatment of dementia and which symptoms are expected to improve

▶ understand the common side effects of dementia medication

▶ understand which investigations are required before and during treatment

▶ know when to seek medical assistance in regards to taking medication.

Keywords

dementia, cognitive function, cognitive impairment, neurotransmitter, side effects, contraindication

---

Introduction

Dementia is associated with a significant and progressive decline in memory, speech, comprehension and the ability to learn new information due to cognitive impairment and is the primary reason for dementia sufferers or their carers to seek medical assistance (Alzheimer's Australia, 2013a). Medications for cognitive impairment can improve memory, alertness and motivation and assist in maintaining independence and living at home for longer. They can also enable people with mild to moderate symptoms to perform activities of daily living (ADLs), as well as complete more complex tasks like shopping and interacting socially (Birks & Harvey, 2006). Medications may slow the decline in the severity of dementia and allow a reasonable quality of life for as long as possible. However, dementia is less responsive to medication in advanced stages due to changes in the chemicals in the brain and damage to the structure of brain cells. Therefore, medications are most beneficial in the early stages and become progressively less effective during the course of the illness.

In addition to cognitive symptoms, people with dementia may also experience behavioural problems such as hallucinations, confusion, aggression, depression, anxiety and insomnia (Alzheimer's Australia, 2013b). These symptoms are usually treated with other medications but the treatment of cognitive and behavioural symptoms has potentially overlapping benefits.

Assessment by a health care professional is required on a regular basis whilst on treatment and carers play an important role in monitoring compliance with treatment and side effects.

What type of doctor/specialist treats dementia?

Many doctors (usually general practitioners) are involved in the investigation and initiation of medications for people with dementia. Following a detailed history, physical examination and relevant investigation, treatment options are then discussed. Specialists such as neurologists, psychogeriatricians, geriatricians and psychiatrists are consulted in difficult cases.

Investigations prior to or during treatment

Before treatment with medication begins, a Mini-Mental State Examination (MMSE) is used in dementia patients as a test to assess baseline cognitive function. It can also be used to monitor the benefits of treatment and the progression of the disease. The MMSE test uses a 30-point scoring system and involves the person completing tasks involving memory and their ability to understand simple commands. Lower scores indicate poorer function (Meade & Bowen, 2005).

No other investigations are specifically required before or during treatment; however, as the majority of dementia sufferers are elderly people (who are prone to infection and illness), blood tests, urine examinations or other investigations may be required from time to time. For example, urinary tract infections (UTIs) cause symptoms that mimic or present as sudden deterioration of dementia and gastroenteritis with diarrhoea and vomiting can cause an electrolyte imbalance increasing the risk of side effects associated with dementia treatments. Investigations are therefore important in identifying if deterioration is due to progression of the dementia or from a concurrent illness.

How often are visits to the doctor required?

Once treatment has commenced, visits to the doctor are recommended every two to three weeks initially and every three to six months when stable. People with associated health problems will be required to consult their doctor more frequently or as suggested by their healthcare team.

How long is treatment required? When is it stopped?

Medication is trialled with the person for six months to see if there is any improvement in cognitive function. The treatment may be stopped at any time if the side effects are too troublesome or if no improvement is seen. The benefit of treatment can be expected to last for about one year. The benefit may not be ongoing as dementia progresses but medications can be continued if there are no contraindications to their use.

What medications are available to treat the cognitive symptoms of dementia?

In Australia, there are two types of medications that are currently available to treat dementia: cholinesterase inhibitors and memantine (Alzheimer's

Australia, 2013c). Both these treatments work on neurotransmitters (chemicals) in the brain and play an important role in the communication between nerve cells. Although the medications themselves cannot cure dementia, they can slow down the course of the disease (Queensland Government, 2012). Medications for treating cognitive symptoms (as well as behavioural symptoms) do, however, have numerous side effects, which include reduced alertness and drowsiness in the initial stages of treatment. The ability to drive may be affected and alcohol intake can mask the benefits of treatment, so both driving and alcohol use should be discussed with the person's doctor. For more detailed information about these medications please refer to the online ancillary chapter at <www.acer.edu.au/living-with-dementia>.

Cholinesterase inhibitors

What are they and how do they work?

Cholinesterase inhibitors (also referred to as cholinergic treatments) are a type of medication used to treat people with mild, moderate and severe dementia. The three main types of inhibitors prescribed are donepezil, galantamine and rivastigmine. These medications work by inhibiting the action of an enzyme called acetylcholinesterase, which destroys a neurotransmitter called acetylcholine. In dementia, memory is affected when the amount of acetylcholine in the brain is reduced and the memory cells start to die. Cholinesterase inhibitors reduce the breakdown of and increase the levels of acetylcholine in the brain (Hill & Briscoe, 2013). This action helps the brain cells to communicate with each other. Improvement in memory, reduction of agitation and reduction in apathy (lack of interest) is noticed after several weeks.

How are they used?

Cholinesterase inhibitor treatments are used once a day to treat dementia. Treatment is commenced at a low dose and gradually increased over four to six weeks to minimise side effects and also to allow time to adjust to the medication and avoid side effects associated with the higher dosage.

Donepezil is one of the more commonly used cholinesterase inhibitors and is available in tablet and dispersible formulations under the names of Arazil, Aricept and Donpesyn. Donepezil is taken at night, ideally at the same time, shortly before going to bed. It can be taken with or without food (Therapeutic Goods Administration, 2008). If a dose is missed, it must be taken as soon as possible but double doses must not be taken.

The second type of cholinesterase inhibitor is galantamine. This type is used widely in Europe and US for the treatment of mild to moderate dementia. As it works in a similar way to donepezil, it has similar side effects and contraindication to use (Allen, 2011)

Rivastigmine is the third type and is also used for the treatment of mild to moderate dementia. It is available as a capsule and liquid for oral use or as a transdermal (skin) patch (Netdoctor, 2013).

Memantine

What is it and how does it work?

Memantine is the most recent anti-dementia medication to be developed and is an alternative type of treatment for people who cannot take cholinesterase inhibitors like donepezil. It works in a different way to the cholinesterase inhibitor treatments and is related to the presence of glutamate. Glutamate is present in high levels in the brain of people with dementia. Memantine blocks the stimulation of a specific receptor that produces glutamate (Allen, 2012). This reduction in the levels of glutamate prevents the brain cells involved in learning and memory from getting damaged.

How is it used?

Memantine is available as tablets and is available under the names of Ebixa and Memanxa. It can be used in people with moderate and severe dementia. Treatment is commenced at a lower dose once a day and is gradually increased over few weeks. Again, this allows time for the body to adjust to the treatment and to avoid side effects associated with a higher dose. It can be taken at any time of day either with or without food; however, it is recommended to be taken at the same time each day to avoid missing any doses (Therapeutic Goods Administration, 2012).

What are the side effects, interactions and contraindication to using cognitive therapies in treating dementia?

Both cholinesterase inhibitors and memantine can interact with other medications. It is therefore advisable to inform the person's doctor and pharmacist if other medicines are being taken concurrently. This includes both prescribed and over-the-counter medications for pain relief, herbal remedies and/or complementary medicines. Side effects are common with both treatments and occur more frequently at a higher dose. However, the effects are generally mild and usually resolve over several weeks if continued. During this period, some side effects can be managed by simple measures. For example, constipation can be managed by dietary changes and increased water intake and headaches can be treated with suitable painkillers.

Cholinesterase inhibitors

Side effects
The most common side effects of cholinesterase inhibitors are nausea, diarrhoea, vomiting, inability to sleep, fatigue, muscle cramps, loss of appetite and weight loss (Hill & Briscoe, 2013). Dizziness and drowsiness may also occur during the first few weeks of treatment.

Interaction with other medications
Cholinesterase inhibitors can interact with other medications. These include:
- over-the-counter medications for allergies, nasal congestion and/or colds
- medications to treat bladder or bowel spasms
- medications, such as aspirin, ibuprofen or naproxen (these can increase the risk of bleeding in the stomach when used with cholinesterase inhibitors like donepezil)
- medications used for anaesthesia (relevant if having surgery).

Concurrent or associated illnesses

Some underlying illnesses may be exacerbated or cause additional problems if used with cholinesterase inhibitors. Although they are not a contraindication to the use of these medications, the person's doctor should be made aware if:

▶ the person has any liver, kidney or heart problems
▶ the person has ever had a stomach ulcer
▶ the person has lung problems, such as asthma or chronic obstructive pulmonary disease (COPD)
▶ the person has a history of seizures (e.g. epilepsy)
▶ the person has ever had an allergic reaction to this or any other medication (Allen, 2011; Alzheimer's Australia, 2013c; NetDoctor, 2013).

Overdose

If a person has taken more than the prescribed dose, medical help should be sought as it can be life threatening. This is advised even if an overdose is suspected but not confirmed. Symptoms of overdose include severe nausea, vomiting, salivation, sweating and convulsions. There are medications that can reverse the effect of these medications but they must be administered as early as possible and in an environment where the person can be monitored. It is advisable to take the prescription bottle with you so that the type and amount of the medication taken can be determined and the severity of the overdose can be assessed.

Memantine

Side effects

The side effects of memantine are generally mild. Common side effects include constipation, confusion, dizziness and headache, drowsiness, insomnia, agitation and hallucinations. Less common side effects include vomiting and anxiety. This medication can also increase muscle tone and sex drive and cause inflammation of the bladder. In rare instances, abnormal body movements called dystonic reactions can occur (Therapeutic Goods Administration, 2012).

Concurrent or associated illnesses

Memantine is contraindicated in patients with epilepsy. However, if the convulsions occurred in the remote past, it may be used with caution. The doctor must be made aware if:

▶ the person has a history of liver or kidney problems

▶ the person has a history of convulsions (seizures, fits or epilepsy)

▶ the person is using any other medicines (Allen, 2012).

Overdose

Overdose with memantine is unlikely to cause serious or life threatening events. However, medical assistance should be sought as it may have serious consequences depending on any underlying health conditions and other medications taken concomitantly. Symptoms of overdose include hallucinations, restlessness, being in a hypnotic state and loss of consciousness. In most cases, a full recovery can be expected.

Medications for behavioural symptoms of dementia

Dementia is associated with behavioural symptoms such as anxiety, agitation, aggressive behaviour, depression, insomnia (sleeplessness), delusions and hallucinations. These can be very distressing for both the person and the carer. These symptoms may be due to illness, changes in the environment or pain (Alzheimer's Australia, 2013b). If underlying illness is excluded, medication may be necessary to treat the symptoms. The possible treatments include major tranquillisers, antidepressants and benzodiazepines.

Medications for treating agitation, aggression and psychosis

Major tranquillisers are used to treat agitation, aggression, delusions and hallucinations. Medications such as haloperidol have side effects such as muscle stiffness, shuffling gait and shakiness even at low doses. Treatments such as risperidone, olanzapine and quetiapine have fewer side effects but may be associated with a small increase in the chance of stroke (Alzheimer's Australia, 2013c).

Medications for treating depression

There are many different medications available to treat depression, most commonly antidepressants. While these treatments can be effective in managing depression reasonably well, simple non-drug interventions, such as an activity or exercise program, can also be of benefit for some people (Alzheimer's Australia, 2013b).

Medications for treating anxiety

Anxiety, panic attacks and extreme or unreasonable fear can be very distressing for the person with dementia (as well as for the carer). Benzodiazepines are very effective for treating anxiety in the short-term. However, patients can become used to their effects and they become less useful with time. Withdrawal can also cause rebound symptoms. These medications can be used for intermittent periods as advised by the person's doctor.

Medications for treating sleep disturbances

Waking at night and night-time wandering can occur in dementia due to confusion from memory loss. Some medications can worsen this as they cause excessive sedation during the day and inability to sleep at night. Increasing activity and stimulation during the day can help. Benzodiazepines should be used as a temporary measure or as a last resort only as they can cause dependence.

Conclusion

As helpful as the current medications to treat dementia can be, unfortunately they do not cure or stop the progression of the disease and not everyone benefits from treatment (Hill & Briscoe, 2013). Medications may, however, slow the decline in mental functions, even if the improvement is temporary and modest (Crouch, 2009).

The choice of medication to use (if any) depends on the individual. There is insufficient evidence that any one medication is more effective but cholinergic treatments are usually considered the first line of treatment. The decision, however, depends upon the side effects, the person's ability to tolerate the medication and contraindication as a result of underlying disease. It is not possible to predict the degree of benefit any one individual will experience with medication.

Early diagnosis of dementia is an important step in the journey as it allows both patient and carer to be involved in treatment choices and plan for the future. Medical opinion should be sought early even if there is only a suspicion of dementia. Although there is insufficient proof, it is possible that earlier intervention with medications may slow down the progression of symptoms.

The treatment of dementia has to be tailored to suit the needs of the individual and requires ongoing monitoring. The need for medication also changes during the course of illness. In the more advanced stages, treatments for behavioural symptoms become more beneficial than improving cognitive symptoms (Alzheimer's Australia, 2013b). The person's general practitioner is in the best position to discuss treatment options and determine if potential benefits outweigh risks associated with medication. Even if temporary, improvement in the quality of life is worth exploring.

References

Allen, H. (2011). *Galantamine*. London: Patient.co.UK. Retrieved from http://www.patient.co.uk/pdf/3829.pdf

Allen, H. (2012). *Memantine*. London: Patient.co.UK. Retrieved from http://www.patient.co.uk/pdf/1421.pdf

Alzheimer's Australia. (2013a). *Help sheet 1: What is dementia?* Melbourne: Alzheimer's Australia.

Alzheimer's Australia. (2013b). *Drugs used to relieve behavioural and psychological symptoms in dementia* [webpage]. Retrieved from http://www.fightdementia.org.au/understanding-dementia/drugs-used-to-relieve-behavioural--psychological-symptoms-of-dementia.aspx

Alzheimer's Australia. (2013c). *Drug treatments and dementia* [webpage]. Retrieved from http://www.fightdementia.org.au/understanding-dementia/drug-treatments-and-dementia.aspx

Birks J., & Harvey, R. J.(2006). Donepezil for dementia due to Alzheimer's disease. *Cochrane Database of Systematic Reviews, 1.* Art. No.: CD001190. doi: 10.1002/14651858.CD001190.pub2

Crouch, A. M. (2009). Treating dementia. *Australian Prescriber, 32*(1), 9–12.

Hill, L., & Briscoe, M. (2013). *Drug treatments in Alzheimer's* [webpage]. London: Royal College of Psychiatrists. Retrieved from http://www.rcpsych.ac.uk/expertadvice/treatments/drugtreatmentofalzheimers.aspx

Meade, C., & Bowen, S. (2005). Diagnosing dementia: mental status testing and beyond. *Australian Prescriber, 28*(1), 11–13.

NetDoctor. (2013). *Rivastigmine* [webpage]. Retrieved from http://www.netdoctor.co.uk/seniors-health/medicines/exelon.html

Queensland Government. (2013). *Choice and medication: Donepezil* [webpage]. Retrieved from http://www.choiceandmedication.org/queenslandhealth/medications/25/

Santacruz, K. S., & Swagerty, D. (2001). Early diagnosis of dementia. *American Family Physician, 63*(4), 703–713.

Therapeutic Goods Administration (TGA). (2008). *Product information (PI) for donepezil.* Retrieved from https://www.ebs.tga.gov.au/ebs/picmi/picmirepository.nsf/pdf?OpenAgent&id=CP-2012-PI-02732-1

Therapeutic Goods Administration (TGA). (2012). *Product information (PI) for memantine.* Retrieved from https://www.ebs.tga.gov.au/ebs/picmi/picmirepository.nsf/pdf?OpenAgent&id=CP-2011-PI-01432-3

Chapter 10

COMPLEMENTARY THERAPIES

Karen Watson
Carrington Centennial Care

Chapter outcomes

When you have completed this chapter you will be able to:

- ▶ understand the role of complementary therapies in different care settings
- ▶ identify which complementary therapies can be administered in home settings
- ▶ appreciate the value of complementary therapies to improve quality of life.

Keywords

aromatherapy, exercise, massage, music therapy, meditation

Introduction

Complementary therapies are enjoyable natural practices that holistically support individual health. Complementary therapies have minimal side effects and interactions and they provide sensory stimulation for people with dementia without overstimulating. When using complementary therapies, reduced incidents of problematic behaviour and increased independence through activities of daily living are reported. Caring for a person with dementia is physically and emotionally demanding. So complementary therapies, when incorporated into a daily routine, support physical, emotional and spiritual health, increasing the quality of life for people with dementia as well as carers.

What are complementary therapies?

Complementary therapies are healing practices that have been used for generations in different cultures throughout the world. Therapies are classified into four domains: biological-based therapies, energy therapies, manipulative and body-based therapies and mind–body therapies. Biological-based therapies use therapies of organic origin and they include aromatherapy, dietary supplementation, herbal remedies and nutrition. Energy therapies influence the energy believed to surround the body through therapies using magnetics, reiki and therapeutic touch. Manipulative and body-based therapies are based in movement, manipulation and bodywork and they include chiropractic treatments, exercise, osteopathy and massage. The last domain of mind-body therapies uses practices aimed to assert the mind's power over body symptoms and they include meditation, music therapy, positive thought and prayer (National Center for Complementary and Alternative Medicine, 2010).

Complementary therapies are not alternatives to medications used by a person to control their condition; they are interventions used concurrently with medications to support treatment and to maintain or improve current levels of physical, emotional and spiritual health. When used correctly complementary therapies have minimal side effects or interactions with western medicines.

While some complementary therapies may take years of practice to master, others can be practised at home safely with minimal training and expense. The equipment used to practise complementary therapies is inexpensive and can be used for multiple sessions. Equipment may include sorbolene cream for massage, CDs or MP3 players for music therapy or guided meditation and essential oils for aromatherapy. Learning about complementary therapies can be fun and rewarding. Print and audio books are available from libraries, information that outlines basic application practice can be found online and correspondence courses may further deepen your knowledge. Once a domain only for qualified practitioners, there is a growing body of research that suggests qualified carers should initiate complementary therapies for the people in their care.

Complementary therapies are often easily implemented in the home and best administered by a carer who has an intimate knowledge of the person with dementia. These therapies may be incorporated into the daily routine or can be strategically implemented when required. The person with dementia may become regularly unsettled in the afternoon and deciding to provide a hand massage at this time might promote relaxation. A walk or therapeutic exercise is best implemented in the morning when the person is alert. A carer will also be aware of when they themselves are becoming overwhelmed by the responsibilities of caring. Carers also need to value their own health as they do the health of those in their care. Diffusing lavender will be enjoyable to both the person with dementia and the carer, promoting wellbeing and self-care.

It is essential that carers be involved in the selection and administration of complementary therapies, as the effectiveness of intervention to some extent is based on the person's individual preferences. A person who does not wish to be touched is not likely to respond to massage, as a person who does not like country music will not respond to that genre of music therapy. A carer who has intimate knowledge of the person with dementia is more likely to have success with natural therapies.

In Australia, 58% of people over the age of 65 have been using complementary therapies within a 12-month period in 2007. Information suggests that Australia's older population is comfortable using, and presumably self-prescribing, complementary therapies within their current medical regimens (Xue et al., 2007). Complementary therapies known to be effective in dementia management include aromatherapy, exercise, meditation, music therapy, massage and therapeutic touch.

Common types of complementary therapies

Aromatherapy

Aromatherapy is defined as the therapeutic use of aromatic plant oils, including essential oils, to provide agreeable scents in living areas. This type of therapy is used to alleviate symptoms such as headaches, stress, digestive problems and insomnia. Scents can be effective due to the specific properties of the essential oils. Lemon balm, for example, shows promising results in lowering anxiety, whilst lavender, when inhaled, has shown to increase quality sleep patterns (Holt et al., 2003). Lavender and lemon balm are commonly used in the treatment of dementia due to their calming and relaxing properties. Research has shown some success in reducing physical agitation, verbal behaviours, wandering and irritation among participants (Ballard et al., 2002; Lin et al., 2007). Aromatherapy's success with minimising aggression may be attributed to the low confrontational application of aromatherapy, as it is incorporated into the surroundings with minimal disruption to routine.

Diluted essential oils can be dispersed in the air by electric diffusers or applied to clothing. The essential oil is inhaled, stimulating the olfactory bulb, which sends impulses to the limbic system in the brain. The limbic system's amygdala governs the emotional response, whilst the hippocampus, located in the cerebral cortex, is involved with retrieval of memories surrounding the scent. It is suggested the limbic system then interacts with the cerebral cortex to control heart rate, blood pressure, breathing, stress and hormone levels (Fontaine, 2011). Essential oils can therefore stimulate or relax people who inhale the essence by triggering happy memories. Aromas of cinnamon, jasmine or mandarin may evoke memories that provide feelings of comfort and security to a person with dementia.

It is important that carers be cautious when using essential oils. Essential oils should never be placed directly on the skin, vaporisers should always be situated in a safe place and, when diffusing oil, always dilute the oil in water (two to three drops in 10 mL of water is the recommended dosage). Be aware that aromatherapy dosage in older people and for palliation is half the dose of that for the rest of the population (Fontaine, 2011).

Exercise

Exercise is a complementary therapy that is necessary to incorporate into the daily routine. It can be disguised as play or activity and the benefits are numerous. Exercise is known to lower blood pressure, increase bone and muscle strength, improve glucose regulation and increase energy levels. Regular exercise can also improve mood, coordination and balance while reducing anxiety and improving sleep patterns. Movement can also increase range of motion by releasing contracted muscles, and mobilising and increasing circulation in the joints. Activities of daily living, such as mobilising, feeding and toileting, can be more easily performed and skills retained for longer (Australian Department of Health and Ageing, 2008).

Exercises should always be tailored to an individual's needs and ability. Walking, if ability permits, can provide stimulation for the mind as well as the body. Other exercises may include simple reaching and clenching movements designed to assist in grasping items such as spoons and combs. A gentle leg lift with ankle rotation will ensure that leg muscles are stretched and blood flow is increased, improving range of motion and flexibility. While functional, exercises should also be enjoyable. For example, balloon tennis and carpet bowls may be used to improve coordination but they may also reignite a passion for an activity once enjoyed.

Two forms of exercise that are commonly used as interventions for people with dementia are therapeutic exercise and adapted tai chi (DeChamps et al., 2010). Therapeutic exercise is a modified exercise program designed for older adults, combining simple upper body movements and resistance training that uses eight to 10 major muscle groups. Sessions are focused on maintaining activities for daily living and can be as little as 10 minutes a day to gain optimum benefit. Adapted tai chi features fewer lower body movements and simpler hand gestures than regular tai chi. There is some support that adaptive tai chi has a positive effect on behaviour management among people with dementia and this may be related to the meditative component during sessions (Dechamps et al., 2010). Both therapeutic exercise and adaptive tai chi require the person to possess the ability to follow simple instructions and mimic the exercises demonstrated; it is therefore not suitable to all stages of dementia.

An initial check-up by a health professional should be obtained before any exercise program begins. Exercises should be relaxed and comfortable and never painful.

Massage and therapeutic touch

Massage can be initiated anywhere along the dementia journey, regardless of ability. However, it becomes especially important in end stage dementia when muscles tend to contract and touch becomes a form of communication. Massage influences soft tissue through pressure, tension, motion or vibration (Australian Association of Massage Therapists, 2007). Massage can reduce blood pressure and heart rate, improving sleep patterns in people with dementia. It also improves anxiety and depression and may assist emotional health in older people. Hand massage is usually performed on older people as it is less invasive than disrobing. It is administered with light, direct pressure to gently and slowly skim the hand's surface, in a stroke known as effleurage; circular motions focusing on the palm can also knead away tensions (Australian Association of Massage Therapists, 2007).

Hicks–Moore & Robinson's (2008) study suggests that massage has a calming effect on the person's body, which may provide comfort reducing agitation. During massage, skin can also be checked for deterioration and lubricants can be applied to maintain skin suppleness and integrity. Light pressure must always be used to protect fragile skin and underlying structures from damage.

Touch is not, however, appropriate for all people with dementia as some find touch too confrontational. In these instances, therapeutic touch may be used. Therapeutic touch is a modality of massage that does not rely on direct physical pressure (Australian Association of Massage Therapists, 2007). This form of massage has also shown promise in having a positive effect on behaviour by promoting relaxation (Woods, Beck & Sinha, 2009).

Music therapy

The music we like to listen to provides us with companionship and defines our individuality. Our preferred music encompasses our culture, beliefs and the way we choose to conduct our lives. It is, therefore, no wonder that it can affect our physiological, psychological and spiritual being. Music therapy has been found to produce a state of wellbeing in an individual when the music is connected to their culture or their preferences (Fontaine, 2011).

Music therapy is the planned and creative use of music to attain and maintain health and wellbeing. It is usually used in a group situation; however, it can be administered alone (Australian Music Therapy

Association, 2006). Music therapy can be conducted with or without singalong. Music is thought to influence specific pathways in the brain associated with emotional behaviours and endorphin release. Endorphins are defined as peptide hormones that are found in the brain and operate as the body's natural painkillers. During activities, like listening to music, these endorphins are released and this can produce feelings of pleasure and a general state of wellbeing (Boso et al., 2006). Music therapy, therefore, has the potential to decrease agitation, verbal behaviours and incidents of wandering. It can also lead to a decrease in anxiety and can improve night–time disturbances. As a carer, taking the time to play a person's favourite music is a celebration of their life.

Guided meditation

Meditation is a personal journey of self-awareness, discovery and reconciliation. People with dementia who participate in meditation are more likely to be involved in group activities and display higher levels of self-esteem. Further, it reduces anxiety and problematic behaviour disruptions among people with dementia and has a positive effect on memory loss and increased brain activity.

Guided meditation is the slowing of the mind to think of nothing but the carer's voice. Reading a guided meditation can prove relaxing and thought provoking for the person with dementia. Meditation usually begins by asking the person to concentrate on their breathing. Once the person is relaxed the carer guiding the meditation then takes them on a journey through storytelling that evokes imagery in the person's mind. The person can mentally leave the difficulties of their reality behind, escaping to a state of bliss and relaxation (Lindberg, 2005). Carers may be able to obtain guided meditation books, CDs and DVDs from their local library or online.

Conclusion

Carers in all settings can initiate complementary therapies, including aromatherapy, exercise, massage, meditation and music therapy. All these therapies appear to be successful in enhancing physical, mental and spiritual health and in supporting the person with dementia and their carer. Aromatherapy and music therapy, in particular, have shown some success in managing physical, aggressive and wandering behaviours. Complementary therapies provide enjoyable relaxing activities for the person with dementia and their carer, strengthening the therapeutic bond and reducing carer stress. The gentle nature and low side effects of complementary therapies support their implementation. Complementary therapies have the potential to alleviate problematic side effects and improve quality of life of people with dementia.

References

Australian Association of Massage Therapists. (2007). *What is massage?* Retrieved from http://aamt.com.au/about-massage/what-is-massage/#content

Australian Department of Health and Ageing. (2008). *Choose health: be active: A physical activity guide for older Australians*. Canberra: Commonwealth of Australia.

Australian Music Therapy Association (AMTA). (2006). *Music therapy: A sound practice*. Malvern, Vic: AMTA.

Ballard, C., O'Brien, J., Reichelt, K., & Perry, E. (2002). Aromatherapy as a safe and effective treatment for the management of agitation in severe dementia: The results of a double blind placebo controlled trial with *Melissa*. *Journal of Clinical Psychiatry, 67*(7), 553–558.

Boso, M., Politi, P., Barale, F., & Emanuele, E. (2006). Neurophysiology and neurobiology of the musical experience. *Functional Neurology, 21*(4), 187-191.

DeChamps, A., Diolez, P., Thiaudiere, E., Tulon, A., Onifade, C., Vuong, T., Helmer, C., & Bourdel-Marchasson, I. (2010). Effects of exercise programs to prevent decline in health-related quality of life in highly deconditioned institutionalized elderly persons. *American Medical Association, 170*(2), 162–169.

Fontaine, K. (2011). *Complementary and alternative therapies for nursing practice* (3rd ed.). New Jersey, NY: Pearson.

Hicks-Moore, S., & Robinson, B. (2008). Favorite music and hand massage: Two interventions to decrease agitation in residents with dementia. *Dementia, 7*(1), 95–108.

Holt, F., Birks, T., Thorgrimsen, L., Spector, A., Wiles, A., & Orrell, M. (2003). Aroma therapy for dementia. *Cochrane Database of Systematic Reviews, 2003*(3). Art. No.: CD003150. DOI: 10.1002/14651858.CD003150. Retrieved from http://onlinelibrary.wiley.com/doi/10.1002/14651858.CD003150/abstract

Lin, P., Chan, W., Ng, B., & Lam, L. (2007). Efficacy of aromatherapy (*Lavandula angustifolia*) as an intervention for agitated behaviors in Chinese older persons with dementia: A cross-over randomized trial. *International Journal of Geriatric Psychiatry, 22*, 405–410.

Lindberg, D. (2005). Integrative research related to meditation, spirituality, and the elderly. *Geriatric nursing, 26*(6), 372–377.

National Center for Complementary and Alternative Medicine. (2010). *What is complementary and alternative medicine?* Retrieved from http://nccam.nih.gov/sites/nccam.nih.gov/files/D347_05-25-2012.pdf

Woods, D., Beck, C., & Sinha, K. (2009). The effect of therapeutic touch on behavioral symptoms and cortisol in persons with dementia. *Forsch Komplementmed, 16*(3), 181–189.

Xue, C., Zhang, A., Lin, V., Da Costa, C., & Story, D. (2007). Complementary and alternative medicine use in Australia: A national population survey. *Journal of Alternative and Complementary Medicine, 13*(6), 643–650.

Chapter 11

MENTAL STIMULATION

Kathryn G Goozee

Anglican Retirement Village

Shona P Nicholls

Anglican Retirement Village

Chapter outcomes

When you have completed this chapter you will be able to:

▸ define the different types of activities, including incidental and planned activities of daily living (ADLs)

▸ influence engagement of the person in activities

▸ understand how the environment influences activity.

Keywords

activities, agreeableness, dementia, environment, meaningful

Introduction

As a carer of someone with dementia, have you ever asked the following question?: 'Is the person under my care bored, in need of more activities or getting enough stimulation?' If this question has crossed your mind, understand that you are not alone. Whether the person with dementia lives within the general community or resides in a residential aged care facility (RACF), most carers share the same concern.

This chapter will provide an overview of why it is important to provide tailored, meaningful activities and how you can enrich the environment, adapt the activities and, most importantly, engage the person. It will offer suggestions for inclusion in the 'activity program' but not dictate which activities must be undertaken. The importance of correctly identifying activities to suit the individual will be highlighted and you will be empowered to plan, adapt, try and try again activities that provide not only stimulation, but offer shared joy and satisfaction in the process.

The importance of activities

Research suggests that providing cognitively stimulating activities to older people is not only beneficial, but adds to a person's general wellbeing and quality of life. Cognitive activity even in later life enhances 'cognitive reserve', which is believed to be protective against developing dementia (Akbaraly et al., 2009; Hall et al., 2009). Valenzuela (2009) emphasises the importance of maximising the use of existing neurons (brain cells) to capitalise on the opportunity to open new pathways. Basically, it is never too late to make a difference.

While it is understood that dementia is a progressive illness, the aim for any activity is to enhance the person's cognition, keep them engaged, provide them with a sense of purpose and generally add light to their day. We know that people with dementia still have healthy brain cells, just fewer of them, so we want to highlight the importance of optimising the functions of those still remaining. To keep the brain cells 'firing' they need to be exercised and stimulated, but not stressed. Stress, which can occur from a poorly planned or poorly conducted activity, can have adverse effects on the behaviour of a person with dementia. People with dementia will often recoil and withdraw from stressful events, thereby impacting on their willingness to participate in activities in the future. Nevertheless, even the most well-planned activities can fail. It is always good to be in tune to the feedback you get by observing the reaction of the person you are taking care of and see if there are any signs of stress. Changing to a different activity with less complexity is one strategy that can help the person to feel at ease.

Engaging interest

Activities are more than just a program to fill the calendar (Kolanowski & Buettner, 2008). When a program is masterfully crafted it offers meaning and pleasure, while providing a blend of familiarity, variety, exploration, fantasy and sensitivity. Quality research is emerging that supports the use of activities in both individual and group settings (Lin et al., 2011; Noice & Noice, 2009). However, different types of dementia can result in people experiencing different cognitive deficits, so activities undertaken still need to be tailored to the individual. They can draw upon a broad range of areas, which may include, but are not limited to, music, art, craft, culture, cooking, gardening, pets, physical exercise, games and social engagement, all of which can stimulate the senses and encourage reminiscence. The right mix of activities should provide each person with a sense of pleasure and contribute to their quality of life, as well as promoting meaningful connections with others. Careful consideration should also be given to ensure that the physical and cognitive abilities of the person (or group) are matched to the task and/or complexity of the activity. Matching individual ability with task complexity increases the likelihood of the person feeling a sense of accomplishment and satisfaction and reduces the risk of them experiencing failure.

Previously enjoyed activities may have already been abandoned, often due to lack of motivation, inability to get to the activity or complexity of the task; however, consider what skills still remain in those areas of interest. Influencing a person's willingness to participate in activities can be one of the biggest hurdles to overcome as, while others see a need, the person with dementia often does not. A lack of willingness or 'agreeableness', as referred to by Hill and Kolanowski (2010), may be a result of a number of factors including their general health, pre-existing personality and dementia, as well as the suitability, type or quality of the activity offered. Other factors that will also influence the outcome include the way in which the activity is presented; the skill of the facilitator; the time and duration of the activity; the number of people participating; the environment; and the complexity of the activity. It all seems very daunting and could discourage you from developing a successful activity but remember: the process of 'doing' and making mistakes needs to be part of the philosophy of the activity.

Finding a meaningful activity

A wealth of information is available on the type of activities that can be offered to the person with dementia, including the Alzheimer's Association's (2010) publication *101 Activities*. Other instructive books are also available (Bell et al., 2007), but be aware that there is no 'one size fits all' solution; we are all individuals and having dementia does not change that fact.

Defining what is meaningful can at times be perplexing, as what is meaningful to one person can be meaningless to another. Also, you need to be aware that meaningful activities are defined differently by different groups of people, such as the person, the carer or family members (Harmer & Orrell, 2008). Even when considering material possessions, this difference can be demonstrated. Things that hold particular relevance or importance to one person can be quickly discounted and unwittingly discarded by another; hence the expression saying 'one person's trash is another person's treasure'. The same logic can be used when considering activities. With this in mind, the key to providing meaningful activities is 'knowing the person'. Offering activities that are known to have been an area of interest or that were previously enjoyed are more likely to be successful; however, do not exclude new and untried possibilities. For example:

A daughter visits her father who is in care. Knowing that he had always enjoyed playing cards, she takes a pack of cards to play 'Patience'. The cards are laid out, and her dad starts to turn over two or three cards. He has lost his ability to recognise the different numbers and types of cards so he begins turning over any card, sometimes matching red to black and other times not even that. Her dad starts to laugh with pleasure. It doesn't matter that he is not playing 'Patience'; they are enjoying a meaningful activity while sharing a special moment.

Utilising information and adapting activities

'Knowing the person' may be less of an effort for family carers, while paid carers will need to rely on information from others. Family or close friends are often only too pleased to provide additional information regarding birth place, past career, hobbies and preference for small or large groups. They can also assist in developing a short life story and providing information about the person's idiosyncrasies and minutiae of daily routine. Creating photo albums or short stories can in itself be an activity, while also providing an avenue for ongoing reminiscence therapy. Remember, when creating albums, or even putting a picture in a frame, place the names of the people in the photo on the picture, so that the person with dementia has prompts for when others enquire. For example:

Marjorie had a large family who all remained very committed to visiting, but she struggled with talking to others about them, as she would mix up names and generations, often referring to her granddaughter as her daughter. The family developed a large poster of their family tree, which enabled each person to add a photo with their name clearly written in large text. When Marjorie mentioned a name, such as Mary, the carer could quickly identify the relationship and also remind her of how they were related. Marjorie always guided visitors to the poster with much pride.

Finding activities for people with dementia is not a secret science; they are the same types of activities that people *without* dementia enjoy. The difference, however, is in the complexity of the task. Remember to break down the activity into 'bite-size' parts.

Reviewing carer expectations

Sometimes it is necessary to adjust the expectations of the carer or person conducting the activity. A major limitation can be created if the carer has concrete views on what the 'outcome' of the activity will achieve. The process of 'doing' and making mistakes needs to be part of the philosophy of the activity. It is not the end result that is important: it is the pleasure of 'doing' that provides the rewards. Rules and boundaries often exist in games or activities, but when people with dementia engage in those activities they are often unable to retain or follow the rules. This means that invariably the rules will be broken and boundaries challenged and the carer must learn to accept the new approach and go with the flow. The case study below is an example of unhelpful and helpful approaches:

> *Mary is a volunteer and has excellent skills in quilt making. She volunteers to run a group for people with dementia. However, Mary finds that some of the group are not capable of even simple stitching of the material. As the participants stitch they miss the layers of material and jumble the fabric. Mary quickly identifies those people who are not doing it correctly and tells them not to touch, only watch, while she continues. This approach is unhelpful and leaves the person with dementia feeling disconnected and possibly useless. An alternative approach may have been to ignore the errors or to give those unable to stitch the task of sorting colours of material or advising on which colours they feel should next be used. This kind of approach can generate warm conversation and laughter, without the person feeling excluded.*

Planned activities do not always work, and when this happens it is easy for the carer to feel disheartened. So much time and effort can go into planning an activity only to find the person with dementia would have preferred to sit in front of the television. It may have been that they were tired, distracted or just wanted to sit and watch the passing parade. Don't give up! What doesn't work this morning might work this afternoon or next week. Sometimes an activity might blossom in different company or with a regular confidante. Don't take it personally. Remember to write down the activities you try, what worked or what may have worked better. Don't keep that information to yourself; share successes and failures so that others can build on your efforts.

Enriching the environment to enhance engagement

Only a relatively small percentage of anyone's day or week is spent on planned activities. A vast amount of time is consumed with activities of daily living (ADLs). Jobs around the home, such as having a shower, getting dressed, making the tea, sorting a cupboard, hanging out the washing, sweeping, making the bed, putting out the rubbish and feeding the pets, are all activities of daily living. Having dementia may not necessarily change the person's desire to do these activities. In fact, a great deal of pleasure can be derived from undertaking them, thus providing a sense of accomplishment at their completion.

Often people with dementia will get restless when they feel they should be doing something. This is commonly seen in the afternoons and referred to as 'sundowning'. What is believed to be happening is an internal desire to 'get organised'. It is the time when everyone returns home, dinner is planned, the house is ordered and night is approaching. If the person with dementia senses this time but does not know what to do, it creates a degree of internal stress. Often these activities have been taken over by the carer, but still the desire to 'get organised' remains. At this time, it is not unusual for the person with dementia to get physically agitated and feel emotionally lost, confused and even very annoyed. They often know that they should be doing something, but don't know how to help or why they are not allowed to help. Therefore, encouraging them to do as much as possible themselves, even if they make errors, will be reassuring. If they cannot engage in an activity at all, try to replace the activities with something else that enables them to feel like they are contributing and therefore maintaining their dignity. An example is described below:

Louisa was an Italian lady who lived in a residential aged care facility and in the evenings became quite restless and difficult to manage. Background information was obtained from her family and it was discovered that Louisa was the youngest of five children and the only daughter. She was described as a caring lady and a mother of two daughters, who previously worked as a cleaner at a large public hospital and had taught herself English. Louisa has also cared for her ageing mother and routinely got up during the night to provide care.

This explained a lot of her current behaviours as Louisa would reposition other residents' feet in bed, pace up and down at night, try to make beds and take the linen trolley.

The staff redesigned her activity program to include more home duty tasks and developed a home corner in the lounge room, complete with dust mop, broom, cups, plates, washing tub and a basket of clean washing. Louisa regained a sense of purpose and her restlessness significantly reduced.

The above example highlights the importance of providing an environment that supports activity involvement. This is generally more easily achieved in a person's own home, compared to a residential facility, but it's not impossible. When looking at the environment, it needs to enable the activity of interest. For example, for the person who has enjoyed woodwork, a workbench may be important; if they sew, a sewing basket and good lighting may be needed.

An enriched environment should incorporate elements of the person's previous home or lifestyle, therefore offering a sense of familiarity and comfort. If relocating to a new address, ensure that the possessions selected for relocation are those things that give meaning. Well-intentioned families will often buy new, colour-coordinated items in an attempt to make the room 'picture perfect'. Old favourites, regardless of their condition or colour, are generally better. A wealth of incidental activity comes with the ornaments, clocks, pictures, bed covers, pieces of familiar furniture, plants, magazines and boxes of oddments. Incidental activity simply refers to unplanned activity that occurs in response to certain objects and the environment. For example, leaving a watering can beside a plant encourages watering, magazines on a table entices reading and a broom against a wall promotes sweeping. Fill the room with cues for incidental, meaningful activity and see what happens.

'Moving objects' is an activity frequently 'underrated' by carers of those with dementia. Possessions will frequently be reported as missing or are found in unusual places. This can be particularly challenging for family members who become engaged in constantly searching for the lost items. However, if you accept that this will happen, sometimes by the person with dementia's own doing or at times by others, the frustration can be reduced. Moving objects is actually a form of incidental activity and while it may cause some frustration at times it is quite a healthy response. A tidy home often lacks opportunity for incidental activity and can increase the person's tendency to interfere with other people's belongings. To reduce carer frustration look for ways to channel this incidental activity by creating a 'busy bench' or an area filled with books, magazines, oddments and the like and encourage the person with dementia to engage. Remember to avoid the temptation of packing everything away to make it all neat and tidy as you are suppressing an opportunity for activity.

While the temptation for carers to 'get the job done' can exist, if a person with dementia wants to help, always try to accommodate them. They may not be able to do it as well or as quickly, or even at all, but give them the chance to help, even in part. For example, you are baking a cake, the ingredients are gathered and the recipe asks for a cup of flour. They could measure the flour, tip the prefilled cup into the bowl, crack the egg, stir in the milk or act as the official taster.

Conclusion

There are a few key tips to consider when venturing out on your quest for the right activity. These include:
► knowing the person
► incorporating activities of daily living and incidental and planned activities into the program
► focusing on the moment rather than the outcome
► matching the ability with the complexity of the task
► breaking down the activity into achievable parts
► considering personal traits and past interests when selecting activities

- ▶ enabling the environment
- ▶ sharing the knowledge
- ▶ not giving up.

The number and type of activities that can be included in your armoury is only limited by your imagination and energy. At times the right activity is nothing at all. Everyone needs downtime (some more so than others), so an extra activity at that time may not be necessary. Spending one-on-one time sitting together, simply holding hands or looking out the window may be all that is needed.

References

Akbaraly, T. N., Portet, F., Fustinoni, S., Dartigues, J.-F., Artero, S., Rouaud, O., Touchon, J., Ritchie, K., & Berr, C. (2009). Leisure activities and the risk of dementia in the elderly: Results from the Three-City Study. *Neurology, 73*(11), 854–861.

Alzheimer's Association. (2013). *101 activities*. Retrieved from http://www.alz. org/living_with_alzheimers_101_activities.asp

Bell, V., Troxel, D., Cox, T., & Hamon, R. (2007). *The best friends book of Alzheimer's activities* (Vol. 1). Baltimore, MD: Health Professions Press.

Hall, C. B., Lipton, R. B., Sliwinski, M., Katz, M. J., Derby, C. A., & Verghese, J. (2009). Cognitive activity delay onset of memory decline in persons who develop dementia. *Neurology, 73*(5), 356–361.

Harmer, B. J., & Orrell, M. (2008). What is meaningful activity for people with dementia living in care homes? A comparison of the views of older people with dementia, staff and family carers. *Aging & Mental Health, 12*(5), 548–558.

Hill, N. L., & Kolanowski, A. (2010). Agreeableness and activity engagement in nursing home residents with dementia: A pilot study. *Journal of Gerontological Nursing, 36*(9), 45–52.

Kolanowski, A., & Buettner, L. (2008). Prescribing activities that engage passive residents. *Journal of Gerontological Nursing, 34*(1), 13–18.

Lin, Y., Chu, H., Yang, C.-Y., Chen, C.-H., Chen, S.-G., Chang, H.-J., Hsieh, C.-J., Chou, K.-R. (2011). Effectiveness of group music intervention against agitated behaviour in elderly persons with dementia. *International Journal of Geriatric Psychiatry, 26*(7), 670–678.

Noice, H., & Noice, T. (2009). An arts intervention for older adults living in subsidized retirement homes. Neuropsychology, development and cognition. *Sec. B: Aging, Neuropsychology and Cognition, 16*(1) 56–79.

Valenzuela, M. (2009). *It's never too late to change your mind*. Sydney: ABC books.

Chapter 12

SPIRITUALITY

Drene Somasundram
Avondale College of Higher Education

Katherine L Cooper
Avondale College of Higher Education

Chapter outcomes

When you have completed this chapter you will be able to:

▸ recognise how spiritual health is interrelated with the body, mind and spirit

▸ understand why spiritual care is important

▸ assess and create a spiritually supportive environment.

Keywords

holism, spiritual needs, spirituality, spiritual assessment, supportive environment

Introduction

Spiritual care has typically been an under-recognised component of care for a person with dementia. Carers may be equipped with the knowledge and skills to provide care for physical and mental needs but leave the spiritual needs unaddressed. This could be because of their unfamiliarity with how to assess for spiritual needs and/or what to do to address these needs once assessed.

This chapter provides an overview of spirituality and the spiritual needs that can arise when a person is faced with living with dementia.

It will offer suggestions of spiritual care methods that the carer can use to provide for the spiritual needs that have been both recognised and assessed. How these strategies can assist the person with dementia to cope with the effects of their disease will be explained so the carer can make informed choices on which methods they choose to provide.

What is spirituality and how does it relate to health?

Caring for a person with dementia not only involves caring for their physical needs, but also their spiritual needs. This is what we call holism; when a person's body, mind and spirit are all addressed (Dossey & Keegan, 2009). Caring that uses a holistic approach incorporates all three of these aspects of care.

In today's contemporary society, there is recognition of the importance of caring for the spiritual needs within health care (Wilding, 2007). Spirituality is identified as an important factor in achieving the balance needed to maintain health and wellness and to cope with illness. It is a force intrinsic to human nature and is one of the deepest and most potent resources for healing. It has been said that 'inherent in the human condition, spirituality is expressed and experienced through living our connectedness with the Sacred Source, the self, others, and nature' (Burkhardt & Nagai-Jacobson, 2013, p. 721).

All human beings have spiritual needs regardless of their world views, faith traditions or cultural context (recognised or not). Spirituality gives an individual a sense of purpose, a sense of forgiveness, the need to love, the need for belief and faith, a sense of mystery, the need for hope and the need to make sense of suffering and death (Crisp & Taylor, 2009). In a multicultural society such as Australia, carers need to be mindful that all human beings have innate universal spiritual needs.

In moments of crisis, and when confronted with actual or potential illness or disability, spiritual needs can surface; although through pain it is not always recognisable. A person asking 'Why me?' stands at a complex junction in their life. Here they question life's meaning and purpose. This spiritual need may cause distress and possibly anger, regret or even guilt, which could drive a person's need for a sense of forgiveness (Crisp & Taylor, 2009). The need for love may express itself in the person wanting to feel safe, have a sense of belonging and to be affirmed and supported by their friends and family. The need for hope is essential to the person who feels threatened by the loss of their independence. Healthcare professionals enter into what O'Brien (2011) calls a privileged, sacred covenant where they enter the person's world and work with them through these tough times.

Why is caring for the spirituality of people with dementia important?

In health care today, a person-centred approach is used to provide care to people with dementia (Keast, Leskovar & Brohm, 2010). This means that the care provided is tailored to the individual needs of each person.

Numerous challenges for carers arise when addressing the spiritual needs of people with dementia. Cognitive deterioration can lead to a decline in the person's ability to perform basic activities of daily living (ADLs). They may experience memory loss, behaviour and personality changes, impaired visual and spatial skills and a decline in the ability to think and recall information (Crisp & Taylor, 2009). People with dementia, therefore, are often unable to articulate or identify their own spiritual needs.

People experiencing dementia suffer debilitating and life-changing symptoms that impact upon their independence. Dependence upon others for routine care can leave the person feeling powerless. This loss of ability to address basic physical needs can impact upon their sense of meaning and purpose and their ability to deal with the changes in function associated with dementia. Those who receive care for their spiritual needs are more likely to successfully adapt to these challenges that arise as the disease progresses (Lindberg, 2005).

We next discuss the three approaches that will aid the carer in addressing the spiritual needs of people with dementia. These are recognising spiritual needs, assessing spiritual needs and providing spiritual care.

Caring for the person's spiritual needs

How do I recognise spiritual needs?

Recognising the spiritual needs of the person with dementia is an important component of providing good spiritual care. Examples include providing a space to pray or the location to pray to Mecca, setting up a shrine with images of their gods and allowing them to use incense.

People with dementia who have their spiritual needs recognised and addressed are more likely to be able to maintain a sense of meaning and purpose, which will enable them to live their life as fully as possible. As the symptoms of their disease progress, they will be able to develop effective coping strategies, make sense of their situation and come to terms with losses related to dementia.

Recognising spiritual needs can also help the person to preserve meaningful connections with the world around them, which will give them a sense of security and belonging. Dependable and meaningful relationships help the person to 'retain emotional responsiveness', 'preserve confidence' and 'assist' in their efforts to engage in life (Keast et al., 2010, p. 4). If the person is religious they may wish to express their spirituality through their religion and continue their relationship with God or another divine being. All this aids in maintaining their quality of life and giving them hope.

How do I assess spiritual needs?

A spiritual history can be difficult for a carer to obtain, as the person with dementia may find it hard to communicate their spiritual needs. If this is the case, the carer should try to find out about any religious practices the person may have by asking their family and friends. If this is not possible, then the carer needs to be able to observe the emotional and physical responses of the person with dementia when they are involved in spiritual activities, such as music and religious services. This will enable the carer to see which spiritual practices provide meaning (Keast et al., 2010). For example, seeing the person with dementia smile and tap their hand to the rhythm when listening to a piece of music may indicate that the music is resonating within them in a meaningful way.

Research shows that assessment of spiritual needs is easier to do when the carer is aware of their own spirituality (Pesut, 2008). In order to be aware of your own spirituality, you need to reflect on what your own perspectives of spirituality are and how these views may affect how you relate to the person with dementia, particularly if your views are different to theirs. This insight will help you to assess and address the person's spiritual needs more effectively.

How can I provide spiritual care?

When providing spiritual care, the carer needs to create an environment that is spiritually supportive. A spiritually supportive environment consists of being physically and emotionally present with the person and showing that you care. The methods listed below can be used by carers to show that they are present in a caring sense. As a carer, you could provide spiritual care by:

▶ holding their hand
▶ hugging them
▶ listening to them
▶ laughing with them
▶ allowing them to talk about their fears and beliefs
▶ being positive
▶ helping them to maintain as much independence as possible
▶ being aware of spiritual practices.

Providing these methods of spiritual care can help confused and disoriented persons to respond better and settle more easily. People with dementia respond particularly well when they sense that the carer is kind and compassionate.

Other ways a spiritually supportive environment can be created is to have photos of family members, friends and pets visible. These photos can be placed in a position where the person can easily see them. The carer can refer to them when spending time with the person with dementia. Remembering what their loved ones mean to them can provide comfort and hope.

Spiritual care can also be provided by taking the person with dementia outside to experience nature. Nature can be a source of spiritual inspiration for some people. Let the person feel the warmth of the sunshine upon their skin, breathe in the fresh air, take in the beautiful sights and smell the fragrances of flowers and scented trees. This can help them feel a sense of peace, and can also help to orientate them to the time of day and season of the year. Taking the person outdoors can result in beneficial spiritual and emotional effects. Even persons with advanced dementia experience less aggression and agitation when this is done (Chalfont, 2008).

When caring spiritually for people with dementia, the carer also needs to consider any religious practices they may have (Curtis & Werthel, 2011). Religious practices may be the means by which the person expresses their spirituality (McSherry, 2007).

In Australia, there is a great diversity of religions with a range of religious practices. Examples of religious practices include:

▶ praying
▶ reading religious books, such as the Bible and Koran
▶ taking communion
▶ attending church
▶ going to confession
▶ listening to music
▶ practising meditation
▶ worshipping to religious shrines.

The carer can spiritually support a person with dementia through their religion by:

▶ providing a quiet time or space if the person wishes to pray or have their family pray with them
▶ respecting a person's religious beliefs, practices and any religious articles such as Rosary beads and religious books
▶ arranging for a chaplain or religious worker associated with their religion to visit
▶ reading to the person from religious books, if requested.

Memory recall exercises can be useful in enhancing a sense of meaning and purpose for the person with dementia. Activities that can be used to prompt memory recall include journal writing and forums. People with dementia can be encouraged to write about experiences in their past and present life. Carers could also help to run forums where groups of people come together to discuss topics relating to what inspires them with hope and faith.

There are other activities that could also help provide a sense of meaning and purpose to the person with dementia. These include encouraging the person with dementia to:

- ▶ garden and take care of pot plants (these activities can help them feel good within themselves)
- ▶ participate in artistic activities such as drawing and painting scenes of nature (these activities can inspire their creative expression)
- ▶ look after a pet (this can be valuable in helping to provide a sense of meaning and purpose, especially as they recall fond memories of pets they have owned in the past).

Spiritual care can also take the form of complementary therapies, which can be used with all people regardless of religious affiliation. Complementary therapies can enhance a person's spirituality and these include:

- ▶ meditation
- ▶ acupuncture
- ▶ reflexology
- ▶ massage
- ▶ colour therapy
- ▶ aromatherapy
- ▶ guided imagery.

Meditation has been found to have particularly beneficial effects among people with dementia. It involves the use of self-enquiry, meditative prayer and imagery. In a study conducted by Lindberg (2005) investigating the effects of meditation upon the older person, it was found that meditation exercises were able to be learned and practised by all people involved in the study, including those who had dementia. The meditation exercises were also found to have a calming effect upon their emotions and behaviour. For more information on complementary therapies see Chapter 10.

Conclusion

People with dementia have spiritual needs. If these needs are addressed with appropriate spiritual care, the person may find the debilitating symptoms associated with dementia easier to cope with. Carers have an important role in providing spiritual care to people with dementia. Carers must recognise that those with dementia have spiritual needs, assess those specific needs and provide spiritual care to suit the individual person.

References

Burkhardt, M. A., & Nagai-Jacobson, M.G. (2013). Spirituality and health. In B. M. Dossey & L. Keegan (Eds.), *Holistic nursing: A handbook for practice* (6th ed.). Sudbury, MA: Jones and Bartlett Publishers.

Chalfont, G. (2008). *Design for nature in dementia care.* London: Jessica Kingsley Publishers.

Crisp, J., & Taylor, C. (2009). *Fundamentals of nursing* (3rd ed.). Sydney: Elsevier Australia.

Curtis, A. M., & Werthel, D. P. (2011). *Religion and healthcare.* Hauppauge, NY: Nova Science Publishers.

Dossey, B. M., & Keegan, L. (2009). *Holistic nursing: A handbook for practice* (5th ed.). Sudbury, MA: Jones and Bartlett Publishers.

Keast, K., Leskovar, C., & Brohm, R. (2010). A systematic review of spirituality and dementia in long term care. *Annals of Long-Term Care: Clinical Care and Aging, 18*(10), 41–47.

Lindberg, D. (2005). Integrative review of research related to meditation, spirituality and the elderly. *Geriatric Nursing, 26*(6), 372–377.

McSherry, W. (2007). *The meaning of spirituality and spiritual care within nursing and health care practice.* London: Quay Books.

O'Brien, M. (2011). *Spirituality in nursing: Standing on holy ground* (3rd ed.). Sudbury, MA: Jones and Bartlett Publishers.

Pesut, B. (2008). Spirituality and spiritual care in nursing fundamentals textbooks. *Journal of Nursing Education, 47*(4), 167–173.

Wilding, C. (2007). Spirituality as sustenance for mental health and meaningful doing: A case illustration. *Medical Journal of Australia, 186*(10), s67–s69.

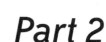

Part 2

UNDERSTANDING HOW TO COMMUNICATE: END OF LIFE AND SELF-CARE

Chapter 13

UNDERSTANDING HOW TO COMMUNICATE

Lenore de la Perrelle
ACH Group

Anne Heard
ACH Group

Chapter outcomes

When you have completed this chapter you will be able to:

▶ identify opportunities to improve communication

▶ implement practical strategies for dealing with common communication concerns

▶ use communication to support the person with dementia.

Keywords

communication, strategies, dementia, respect, support

Introduction

> *… it is important to give us time to collect what is left of our thoughts, and the time to find the words to tell you about them (Swaffer, 2011, p. 19).*

The words of a person living with dementia remind us that dementia presents us with a human problem, and it is at the human level that we find solutions to communicating with people with dementia in a way that we would want for ourselves.

Communication is at the heart of these human solutions, and learning how to improve carers' communication with people with dementia is the focus of this chapter. It is also the focus of much of the literature on person-centred dementia care. Early work by Professor Tom Kitwood and Buz Loveday (1998) in Bradford, United Kingdom, advocated 10 key principles of person-centred care to focus on the person, rather than dementia, as the key to improving care (see Table 13.1).

Table 13.1 Ten key principles of person-centred care

1. Attend to the whole person	2. Each individual is unique
3. Respect the past	4. Focus on the positive
5. Stay in communication	6. Nourish attachments
7. Create community	8. Maximise freedom
9. Don't just give, receive as well	10. Maintain a moral world

Source: Loveday & Kitwood, 1998

At the centre of these principles is communication. It is what sets humans apart from all other beings and is the key to our social existence. We maintain and develop relationships and roles through communication, so when dementia limits and complicates communication it is not surprising that carers and people with dementia experience difficulties in relating to each other.

The two main types of communication problems caused by dementia that Loveday and Kitwood (1998) have identified are:

1. **The carer cannot understand what the person with dementia is trying to communicate.** This can be due to a range of physical conditions such as hearing or visual impairment, or aphasia; a language impairment; or due to difficulty actually speaking due to stroke or muscle weakness (South West Yorkshire Mental Health NHS Trust, 2008).

2. **The person with dementia cannot understand what the carer is trying to communicate.** This can be due to the speed with which they speak, making it difficult for the person with dementia to process the words; the background noise; or complicated speech that overwhelms the person.

This chapter focuses on understanding the perspective of the person with dementia, to improve carers' understanding of what they are trying to communicate and the challenges they face. It then provides ways to improve carer communication so that the person with dementia can better understand what they are trying to get across.

The assumptions that we adopt in offering these strategies are that:

▸ the person with dementia is doing their best to understand us, given their remaining skills and the progression of their cognitive losses

▸ the person's abilities to communicate vary over time and with changes in their health and the social environment we create

▸ improvements in communication can only happen if we learn to create positive environments for communication and develop new communication skills

▸ it is our responsibility to do this as the person with dementia cannot (Loveday & Kitwood, 1998).

The evidence base that we use includes:

▸ interviews with people with dementia and published biographies to identify their perspectives

▸ interviews with carers and published stories to identify the concerns they highlight

▸ person-centred care literature and recent research from Australia and overseas on communication strategies to assist understanding and empathy (this approach reinforces the person-centred approach to care and communication as the key to improved relationships).

We first consider the context of communication for the person with dementia, for the carer and the setting of care to identify the elements that can enhance communication or cause difficulties. By recognising the impact that dementia has on the ability to communicate and understand, we identify how to adapt both the process and the content of communication to improve understanding.

We then offer communication strategies based on the language of respect, inclusion, humour, empathy, touch and silence as a way of developing and maintaining relationships, inclusion in social situations and maintaining dignity and control for the person with dementia through the whole journey. Practical examples and tips for dealing with common communication concerns are provided from the perspective of the person with dementia, the family carer and the careworkers who provide support.

The context of communication for the person with dementia and their carer

The setting in which communication is occurring is an essential element of communication. It is not just the words and the way you communicate; it also matters where you communicate (see Figure 13.1). Professor Tom Kitwood's person–centred approach to dementia care was developed through observations of the impact of the context of care on personhood (Kitwood, 1997). The setting and the feeling of the place can affect communication and meaning. Consider the difference in the communication in a person's own home, at a shopping centre full of noise or in a formal care environment. The familiarity, the established roles, the sense of control and meaning of the person's home is threaded through the communication. At a shopping centre, the noise and stimulation can fatigue or overwhelm a person with dementia, shutting down communication. In an aged care facility communication may be more formal, task-focussed and can highlight the sense of changed relationships and roles.

Christine Bryden talks of a 'knowing' in relationships that goes beyond remembering names or times spent together with family or friends. It emphasises the difference between intimate communication and the more functional discussion about tasks or activities of daily living.

I treasure your visit as a 'now' experience in which I have connected spirit to spirit. I need you to affirm my identity and walk alongside me. I may not be able to affirm you, to remember who you are or whether you visited me (Bryden, 2005, pp. 110–111).

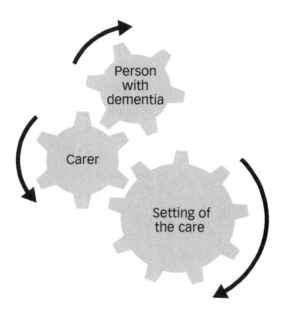

Figure 13.1 Communication related to the setting and relationships

Dawn Brooker's framework of care, putting into practice the person-centred approach, also emphasises the context of care. She identifies the effect of the social environment as another key ingredient of care (Brooker, 2007). How people relate to each other depends to some extent on the feel of the setting. Does it have a feel that the person with dementia is in control of the care or is there a focus on getting tasks done? Is there one way of doing things for all or is care personalised to suit the preferences of the person with dementia? McCormack links the place or setting of care and the sense of self that is supported by the place we inhabit as important elements of relationships (McCormack, 2004).

The common link through this focus on the person in relationships with others is communication. How we interact with each other, our roles and the setting can affect communication.

> *Busy shopping centres are much less accessible to me, as I find them simply exhausting, with loud 'muzak', tills ringing, people talking, children crying. Even a quiet shopping trip can be very stressful if I go with someone, and*

am expected to hold a conversation as well as cope with shopping decisions and the sights and sounds around me (Boden, 1998, p. 68).

The perspective of the person with dementia

People with dementia are individuals and don't necessarily respond in the same ways. For the person with dementia, communication can be affected by the progress of the condition, through other health-related effects, their own personal style, their relationships with others, their experiences in their life and the way the care is offered. There can be changes in the person's level of functioning, and therefore their ability to communicate, as the disease progresses, but there can be fluctuations from minute to minute, hour to hour, day to day. The person may be quite lucid at one time and appear very confused at another.

In my present condition there are times when I feel normal. At other times I cannot follow what is going on around me as the conversation whips too fast from person to person and before I have processed one comment the thread has moved to another person, or another topic and I am left isolated from the action – alone in a crowd (Davis, 1989, p. 85).

The effect of dementia on communication

Dementia is a term for a range of conditions and can affect a person differently according to the cause of dementia, the progress of the condition and the interaction with other health conditions.

For some people with dementia, short-term memory is lost early; others lose inhibition, planning or words earlier. For people for whom English is not the first language, dementia may bring a loss of English and the use of their first language for communication. For some the meaning of words changes significantly.

Sometimes I see words in a strange way, not as whole words but as if they had been split in two … Words become scrambled or lose their meaning (Swaffer, 2011, p. 17).

The effect of other health conditions on communication

Other health conditions can affect the progress of the condition and the ability to communicate. Loss of hearing or vision can have a big impact on a person who is also losing their ability to process conversations. Anxiety or depression can also amplify the impact of dementia on communication, while vascular disease, pain and infections can cause confusion and detract from the ability to make sense of the communication.

Personal reaction to the diagnosis of dementia

For most people, the diagnosis brings shock and despair at the prospect of loss of abilities and lack of treatments or cure. Many people experience a sense of grief and related depression at having to deal with this condition and withdraw from relationships and day-to-day life.

> When I was first diagnosed in 2008, the tears ran down my cheeks non-stop for almost three weeks (Swaffer, 2011, p. 17).

The individual style of the person and their unique personality, will affect communication. Some people are more introspective, tuning into their own thoughts as they monitor the effects of dementia on their communication. This can make it appear that the person is not interested in communication, or that they are unable to do so. Others spend considerable energy covering up their difficulty with communication to avoid embarrassment or avoid conversations for fear of showing their incoherence. Cultural differences, such as beliefs about dementia, or the terms used to describe dementia can alter how willing a person is to discuss how they are feeling or to ask for assistance. Carers who are in a hurry, don't know the person well or who miss the cultural communication cues may mistake individual style for inability to communicate. Some may dismiss symptoms or minimise the effects when the person may feel very strongly about their losses.

The perspective of the carer

Professor Henry Brodaty, a leading specialist in dementia care in Australia, sees the family caregivers of people with dementia as critical to the quality of life of the care recipients. There are some positive outcomes to caring. A sense of love, fulfilment and a reciprocal bond are the chief reasons given for being a caregiver for a spouse or parent (Brodaty & Donkin, 2009). Careworkers are also motivated by what they can offer to support a person to live well. However he also sees high levels of burden for caregivers dealing with grief, fatigue, overload and a sense of being trapped in the role (Brodaty & Donkin, 2009). A recent pilot study reports that up to a quarter of family carers can also experience thoughts of suicide when feeling overburdened in their role (O'Dwyer et al., 2013). Communication is deeply affected when the carer is exhausted, isolated and unsupported. It is hard to maintain a loving tone of voice when answering the same question about what day it is, for the fifteenth time that day, when the carer is also undertaking all the tasks in the home and grieving for the lost relationship with their family member. The key to improving communication for carers is increasing knowledge, self-efficacy and gaining support.

Adapting the process and content of communication: some practical strategies

A range of strategies and practical tips for communication can be best remembered through the principles of respect, inclusion, empathy, touch, humour and silence (see Figure 13.2). These act as a way of checking both the content and the process of the communication, remembering the perspective of the person with dementia, the perspective of the carer and the setting of communication. These principles can form the language of communication with a person with dementia and can help to develop and maintain relationships.

The language of respect

The essence of good communication is mutual respect, having an understanding of, and empathy for, the person's experience and a commitment to optimise the abilities the person still has. This allows the person to maintain their dignity and sense of identity and ensures the wellbeing of both parties.

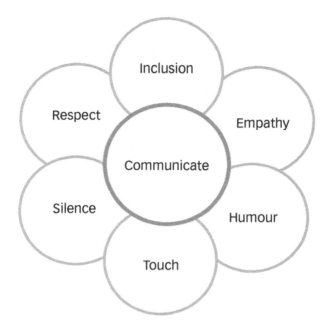

Figure 13.2 The language of communication

Respect for the person as a unique individual

A person enters the experience of dementia with a history of meaningful life experiences, achievements and relationships that have shaped their attitudes, values and personality. It is important to respect that the same person is still present in a changed, but not lesser, capacity. In this way, you acknowledge the worth of that individual and the significance of their life.

You set the tone of communication with your approach. Your words and body language need to reflect a genuine regard for the 'essence' of the person, their 'personhood'.

Respect for the symptoms of the condition

It is difficult to know how much the person with dementia understands. The process of communication is very complex and affected by the nature and extent of damage in the person's brain. They may appear to be listening to what you are saying but not be able to process the information. However, you cannot assume that because the person is not responding that there is no understanding. The person may be processing what you are saying but not be able to work out what to say or do in response. They may know how they want to respond but may not be able to initiate or deliver the response to form the words or action. It is not respectful to talk about the person, or over the person, as if they are not there.

Gaining attention

People with dementia can find it difficult to concentrate and can become easily distracted.

> *It feels as if there is cotton wool in my head, a sort of fog over my thoughts and feelings. This fog means it is hard to focus, to pay attention, and keep up with what is going on around me (Bryden, 2005, p. 106).*

Tips for gaining the person's attention

Before addressing the person it is important to gain their attention. Carers can do this by:

- using the person's name
- approaching the person from the front
- identifying themselves and starting the conversation socially (e.g. you could say 'Mary, it's Jane. How are you today?', wait for a response, then say 'I've come to help you with your shower.')
- using direct eye contact – keep your eyes at the same level as the person so as not to appear threatening
- reducing distractions (e.g. ask if you might turn down the TV or radio, or move into a quiet area)
- avoiding the need to shout from another room as this can be confusing.

Reminding the person of names

People with dementia often lose names first, including the names of people they know.

> *I know faces and know that I connect with them somehow, but not why I know them and what I know about them (Bryden, 2005, p. 109).*

Tips for reminding the person of names

To assist the person in remembering names carers can:

▶ introduce themselves as they greet the person (e.g. 'Hi, Mum, it's Mary, your daughter.')

▶ use prompts and reminders, such as name tags or labels or by using prompting questions (e.g. 'Do you mean ...? or 'Are you looking for your glasses?')

Simple communication

People with dementia may not be able cope with more than one piece of information or instruction at a time. They can become easily overwhelmed.

Tips for simple communication

To help make it easier for the person to communicate carers should:

▶ give one comment or idea at a time

▶ keep instructions short, simple and clearly stated

▶ break instructions down into small steps – give one step at a time

▶ demonstrate routines

▶ allow time for a response

▶ check for understanding

▶ reconsider the complexity and pace of what you are saying (if the person does not understand)

▶ repeat instructions in the same words (rewording the instructions provides additional information for the person to process).

Orientation and instructions

People with dementia may forget instructions and not understand what you expect them to do. They may say 'Yes' and then not act as you have asked. They may need reminding over and over again about things that others remember after one instruction.

> *It is harder to process information, to know how to act and respond, how to behave appropriately and know what to do in everyday situations.*

There are ... moments when slips of my tongue or mind are evident, and I struggle with the effort of finding the right words (Swaffer, 2011, p. 17).

Tips to help with orientation and instructions

To help the person with dementia with orientation and instruction carers should:

▶ explain simply why they are there and what they need to do
▶ make instructions sound clear if they are important or urgent (e.g. 'Stop now', 'Sit there' or 'Hands on the table; now sit')
▶ talk less, demonstrate more
▶ check for understanding.

Slowing communication

People with dementia can be slow to respond as the messages find pathways around the damaged areas of the brain.

Speed is absolutely impossible. Just forget about speed. We're not going to be fast remembering things and knowing things and doing things. When someone wants me to hurry up, I can't hurry up — there's no way to hurry up (Henderson, 1998, p. 79).

In the busyness of caring responsibilities it is easy to become focussed on the task at hand and communicate urgency to the person with dementia. This urgency can be communicated in the pace and tone of your speech, your gestures and body language as impatience, frustration or 'bossiness'. It can cause the person to feel anxious, confused or startled. These feelings can lead to distressed, resistive and sometimes aggressive behaviour. The task can then take longer to be completed.

Tips to responding to slowed communication

Carers can respond to slowed communication by:

▶ using a calm, gentle approach
▶ matching their speed to the person with dementia — slow down!

▶ allowing time for a response – silently count to five
▶ prompting when needed.

Continuing the communication

People with dementia may be unable to say exactly what they want to say or can lose their train of thought as the messages get blocked in the brain.

> … *Don't interrupt our thread of thought, but let us interrupt you when an idea comes into our head, because if we wait, it will disappear … Give us time to speak, wait for us to find the word we want to use, and don't let us feel embarrassed if we lose the thread of what we say (Bryden, 2005, p. 139).*

Tips for continuing the communication

To enable the person to keep their train of thought carers should:
▶ allow time for a response
▶ repeat a word or phrase that has been said to provide a prompt (e.g. 'You were telling me about …')
▶ prompt with 'Do you mean …?'
▶ try to find the meaning implied if the words are not clear.

Repeated questions

People with dementia may repeat questions, statements or stories.

> … *we will ask the same question again without any awareness that we have asked it before. And we need to ask you questions to address our anxiety about an issue … Yes, it does drive you crazy to hear the same thing over and over, but how much worse is it for the person with dementia who knows they have asked you a question but don't remember your answer? (Bryden, 2005, p. 107)*

Depending on where in the brain the damage is, this repetition may be because:
▶ they have forgotten that they have asked or told you before

▸ once started they may be unable to stop and move onto a different topic of conversation.
▸ they are confused or anxious and are seeking information or reassurance (e.g. 'What am I supposed to be doing now?').

This can be very frustrating for the carer, but it is important to respect why this is happening.

Tips on handling repeated questions

To avoid frustration and anxiety carers should always try to:
▸ respond to the question or story as if it is the first time you have heard it
▸ respond to the feelings they are expressing (e.g. 'You seem a bit worried. It's almost dinner time. Would you like to come and help me set the table?')
▸ rephrase the question with empathy (e.g. 'I know you like to be organised ...')
▸ rephrase the question with a related reminiscence (e.g. 'getting ready for dinner was always a busy time')
▸ listen for the feelings, tone and symbols in the question rather than just the question.

Written language

> Reading's almost impossible. For one thing – things don't stand still. Words don't stand still. It appears to me that it's wavering. I can't pin it down – the words – they can be over yonder and over yonder and I can't catch them ... I can see the words, I can pronounce the words, but they don't seem to mean a whole lot (Henderson, 1998, p. 23).

Written prompts and reminders can be helpful for some people with dementia, particularly early in the illness. A larger size and simpler style of font can assist a person to continue to read. Some people find using technology helpful in recording information or reminders and then reading them to reinforce their memory or knowledge (Taylor, 2007).

Tips for using written language

To help the person with reading carers can:

▶ check the person's ability to read the font and understand what is written

▶ encourage the person to use technology, calendars, diaries and written notes as reminders

▶ label places for keys, or put names or pictures on doors to show locations, such as the toilet or where to find cups or food

▶ use name tags to help the person recognise them or use their name in a conversation.

The language of inclusion

A person with dementia may be unable to plan and organise and can often have difficulty making decisions. However, including the person in the process can support their sense of self and understanding.

> *If you take over our lives, then it is so easy for us to withdraw into helplessness (Bryden, 2005, p. 103).*

> *Many decisions are simply so complex and I can't remember what has been said or offered so can't decide. It is much easier to 'go with the flow' (Bryden, 2005, p. 102).*

It is so easy and often quicker to make decisions for people with dementia. However, this diminishes their sense of control over their life, lowers their self-esteem and threatens their identity and the remaining abilities they have.

The challenge then is how to communicate alternatives to the person with dementia, being respectful of their abilities and taking their special communication needs into account

Tips for offering choice

To help the person with dementia feel included but not overwhelmed carers can:

▶ limit choices (e.g. 'Would you like to sit in this chair [pointing] or this one?')

▶ use non-verbal prompts – hold up or point to choices
▶ ask questions that can be answered with a 'Yes' or 'No' – open-ended questions can be confusing and overwhelming (e.g. 'Would you like a cup of tea?' rather than 'What would you like to drink?')
▶ use statements to give information to assist in the decision-making (e.g. 'Would you like the fish? You enjoyed the barramundi last time we came.').

Brackey (2007) describes the concept of the 'illusion of choice' in which a person with dementia who is unable to make decisions is guided in their choice. Instead of asking 'What would you like to wear today?', hold up two outfits and ask 'Which one would like to wear? The blue one or the red one?' If the person is still not able to make a decision, give them a reason to choose one of the outfits. 'I like the blue dress. It brings out your beautiful blue eyes.' This gives an illusion of choice at the same time as taking the opportunity to acknowledge the qualities of the person.

People with dementia often withdraw from social situations as they lose their confidence and abilities to initiate and maintain conversation. They can become increasingly isolated.

> *In my mind, one of the most important things you can do for me to feel comfortable in a group of people is to include me. Not so much by asking questions, unless you're willing to answer them (which I would appreciate) but by including me in your smiles and eye contact ... I don't have as much to contribute to the conversation, but I love being equally included (Simpson & Simpson, 1999, p. 123).*

Tips for inclusion

To help the person feel included in social situations carers can:
▶ include the person in the middle of the group so they can be easily gathered into the conversation with smiles, eye contact and prompts
▶ make a statement, followed by a Yes/No question – this can assist the person to participate (e.g. 'Tom, we really enjoyed that fishing trip on the Murray, didn't we?')

▶ address the person by name and give them direct eye contact – this gains their attention and invites them into the conversation.

The language of humour

Even people with advanced dementia can respond to humour. Respectful humour can lift spirits and diffuse tense situations for both you and the person with dementia.

Humour can be exchanged not only through words but also through facial expressions and gestures.

Tips for using humour

To help lighten the mood carers should:

▶ get to know the person, their unique sense of humour and what makes them laugh
▶ seize appropriate opportunities to add humour to the conversation
▶ respond to the person's expressions of humour, even if confused
▶ laugh with the person, not at them
▶ validate the laughter (e.g. 'we had a good laugh about that' or 'that really tickled your funny bone')
▶ use a familiar saying about laughter, appropriate to the person's culture.

The language of silence

So often when you are with people with dementia you may be tempted to provide answers, and ask questions in an attempt to assist the person to converse or to get them to do what you want them to do. Silence can be uncomfortable. However, filling the space with words might not allow the person the chance to respond or can be overwhelming and confusing. Silences can also offer opportunities to observe what might be happening for the person and to consider your most appropriate response. This is illustrated by a person with dementia in a poem quoted by John Killick (Killick & Craig, 2012, p. 199):

... Words can make or break you.

Sometimes people don't listen,

they give you words back,

and they're all broken, patched up.

People with dementia invite you to be 'present' with them, to be comfortable in the silence and to give your full attention to them.

Tips for being present

To be fully present with the person with dementia carers should:

- listen attentively to what the person is saying or expressing
- look for meaning behind words
- listen to the non-verbal communication: frowns, smiles, sighs and gestures
- allow pauses
- just be with the person: smile, look at them, touch their hand or look at something together
- use gestures or sighs instead of words.

The language of empathy

People with dementia can experience frustration and distress as they try to make sense of an increasingly confusing world and experience a loss of control over their lives.

> *You know when you lean back on a chair and you almost fall over backward, but you catch yourself at the last second, and you don't fall? Do you know that feeling? ... I feel that way all the time (Rose, 1996, p. 105).*

It is important to accept and understand the need being expressed and respond appropriately. Help the person to express their feelings in their own unique way. Their words may be confused but their body language and gestures may clearly express what they are feeling.

> *As our thoughts and words are tangled and confused, you will need good listening skills, being attentive to non-verbal cues ... Don't correct us, just try to understand the meaning of what we intend to say (Bryden, 2005, p. 139).*

Tips for using empathy

When the person seems frightened, distressed or anxious carers should:

▶ stop what they are doing and sit or stand with the person

▶ give direct eye contact

▶ listen attentively, even if their words don't make sense – the act of listening communicates concern and interest

▶ use reassuring words, phrases and body language

▶ acknowledge the emotions they are expressing (e.g. 'You seem really worried/sad ...')

▶ seek reasons for the feelings being expressed – use Yes/No questions (e.g. 'Is your leg hurting?' or 'Are you looking for ...?')

▶ provide opportunities for the person to talk about how they are feeling, if they would like to or are able to.

Unrealistic questions

A person with dementia often has a different perception of reality as recent memories are lost and those from the past become more readily recalled. It is common to hear people with dementia say 'I want to go home' or 'Where is my mother?', which can seem illogical and unrealistic. These can indicate disorientation in time and space, and them 'living in the past'. For the person in their confused state, this is their reality. Arguing with the person or pointing out the present reality can only make them feel more distressed and agitated.

Instead, consider the needs and feelings being expressed in these statements. They could be expressions of their insecurity, of wanting to go back to a time where everything made sense and they felt safe and secure. You may attempt to meet these needs for comfort and security through reminiscence, so that they can relive some of the memories of that relationship or give reassurance that they are in a safe place and cared for. Gentle reorientation may develop in the conversation or the person may realise that it was in the past.

Tips for dealing with unrealistic questions

When confronted with unrealistic questions carers should:

▶ not confront the person with the present reality

- if the person wants to go home, engage the person in conversation about their home
- engage the person in a valued activity (e.g. the person can be invited to have a cup of tea while they are waiting)
- if the person asks 'Where am I?', remind them where they are, the time and occasion (e.g. 'You are at my place and we are having a coffee before we start the dishes')
- if the person asks 'What am I supposed to be doing?', give clear instructions about what you would like them to do (e.g. 'Sit here while I put on the kettle' or 'We are waiting for our turn with the doctor').

Recalling past experiences

Acknowledging the person's reality through reminiscence can be a meaningful way of communicating with a person with dementia. Engaging with people in conversations about their past life experiences can build rapport, reinforce the person's identity, acknowledge their wisdom and learning and heal loneliness and isolation.

Tips to make the most of the person's abilities to recall past experiences

To make the most of the abilities that the person has to recall past experiences carers can:

- use photographs, personal items, memorabilia, books and magazines as reminiscence prompts
- consider what they've learnt about the person and seize opportunities to engage in conversation with them
- sing the person's favourite song while they are assisting them – this shows the person that the carer knows what they like and that they are familiar.

Non-verbal communication

People with dementia may lose the ability to make sense of your words but may 'tune in' to non-verbal communication (your body language, gestures and tone of voice).

Tips for using non-verbal communication

Non-verbal communication that carers can use includes:

▶ a handshake, which is a common greeting in many cultures and shows respect

▶ a gesture with a hand, which may indicate what the carer wants them to look at and prompts the person to do what is needed

▶ a sigh, which can show relaxation or contentment

▶ a shrug of the shoulders, which can show that the carer doesn't know

▶ a matching facial expression to the emotional state to show congruity (a smile when someone is upset may be confusing)

▶ a smile – it only takes a moment and can communicate caring, and inclusion.

The language of touch

> *... this fact that we live in the present, with a depth of spirit and some tangled emotions, rather than cognition, means that you can connect with us at a deep level through touch, eye contact, smiles (Bryden, 2005, p. 99).*

Touch can be an important way to communicate with people with dementia, particularly as words lose their meaning and life becomes overwhelming. As well as communicating instructions, respectful touch can communicate empathy and reassurance. Not everyone, however, will be comfortable in being touched. Some may misinterpret the gesture and respond aggressively or with fear and confusion.

Tips for using touch to communicate

When using touch to communicate carers should:

▶ get to know the person and their level of comfort in regard to being touched

▶ ask if touch is appropriate for the person

▶ use gentle touch to gain attention, give direction or provide comfort and reassurance

▶ note the person's response to touch

▶ consider using touch towards the end of life – gentle massage and touch on the hands, face or hair can be very comforting.

Conclusion

In attempting to communicate with people with dementia, it is important to always consider the nature of the relationship and the context of your communication. If we, as carers, adopt the perspective of the person with dementia we gain greater insights into their difficulties and feelings and can make the adaptations needed to be able to continue to communicate in some way with the person throughout their journey. They are still a person struggling with a condition out of their control. It is the responsibility of the carer to adapt to the changing communication needs as their condition progresses. While the demands of caring for a family member or for a client (if you are a careworker) can be onerous at times, it is always important to assume that the person is doing their best to communicate with us. Where long-standing family patterns make caring particularly difficult, it is important to seek support so that you can maintain your relationship with the family member and not burn out.

When using language the key questions carers should ask include the following:

▶ What language am I communicating? It is good to be conscious of how you are presenting yourself to the person.

▶ Is this the language of respect for the person, for the effect of the disease on the person, for their unique personality and their culture and language?

▶ Is this the language of inclusion of the person in the family or group, in a conversation or in a social setting?

▶ Is this the language of humour? Enjoy a sense of fun with the person, not at their expense.

▶ Is this the language of silence? Be with the person, allowing pauses and non-verbal communication to say it all.

▶ Is this the language of empathy? Can I listen to the feelings behind the words or actions? Am I able to see things from their perspective or just from mine?

▶ Is this the time for the language of touch? Can I bring comfort through gentle touch? Can I show that I am there with the person without the complication of words?

The opportunity to continue to communicate with a person with dementia throughout their journey is there. Wonderful moments can be shared and a deep sense of relationship can be experienced that makes us truly human. It remains our responsibility to adapt our communication to meet their needs.

References

Boden, C. (1998). *Who will I be when I die?* Sydney: Harper Collins Publishers.

Brackey, J. (2007). *Creating moments of joy: A journal for caregivers.* West Lafayette, IN: Purdue University Press.

Brodaty, H., & Donkin, M. (2009). Family caregivers of people with dementia. *Dialogues in Clinical Neuroscience, 11*(2), 217–228.

Brooker, D. (2007). *Person-centred dementia care: Making services better.* London: Jessica Kingsley Publishers.

Bryden, C. (2005). *Dancing with dementia.* London: Jessica Kingsley Publishers.

Davis, R. (1989). *My journey into Alzheimer's disease.* Wheaton, IL: Tyndale House Publishers.

Henderson, C. S. (1998). *Partial view: An Alzheimer's journal.* Dallas, TX: Southern Methodist University Press.

Killick, J., & Craig, C. (2012). *Creativity and communication in persons with dementia.* London: Jessica Kingsley Publishers.

Kitwood, T. (1997). *Dementia reconsidered: The person comes first.* Berkshire, UK: Open University Press.

Loveday, B., & Kitwood, T. (1998). *Improving dementia care: A resource for training and professional development.* London: Hawker Publications.

McCormack, B. (2004). Person-centredness in gerontological nursing: An overview of the literature. *International Journal of Older People Nursing, 13*(3a), 31–38.

O'Dwyer, S., Moyle, W., Zimmer-Gembeck, M., & De Leo, D. (2013). Suicidal ideation in family carers of people with dementia: A pilot study. *International Journal of Geriatric Psychiatry.* doi: 10.1002/gps.3941

Rose, L. (1996). *Show me the way to go home.* Forest Knolls, CA: Elder Books.

Simpson, R., & Simpson A. (1999). *Through the wilderness of Alzheimer's: A guide in two voices.* Minneapolis, MN: Ausburg Fortress Press.

South West Yorkshire Mental Health NHS Trust. (2008). *Dementia toolkit.* Retrieved from http://www.southwestyorkshire.nhs.uk/documents/832.pdf

Swaffer, K. (2011, September). My unseen disappearing world. *The Big Issue,* 16–19.

Taylor, R. (2007). *Alzheimer's from the inside out.* Baltimore, MD: Health Professions Press.

Chapter 14

UNDERSTANDING HOW TO CARE FOR THE DYING

Linda Ora
Nepean Blue Mountains Local Health District

Chapter outcomes

When you have completed this chapter you will be able to:

▸ understand what is meant by 'end stage dementia' and how a 'palliative approach' guides care and decision-making at the end of life

▸ appreciate the importance of advance care planning in the early stages of the disease to assist with end-of-life preferences for treatment and care

▸ recognise the physical signs of dying, understand why they are occurring and how to provide comfort to the person

▸ understand what to do after the person has died and explore the effect grief may have on the carer.

Keywords

end stage dementia, palliative approach, advance care planning, bereavement, dying

---

Introduction

It is a difficult and sad reality, but dementia is an incurable and terminal illness. The person with end stage or advanced dementia is fully dependent on others for all aspects of living. The caregivers, therefore, are central to the quality of life for the person dying from dementia. This chapter has been written to help carers understand the process of dying and describes what carers can do when the goal of care shifts from cure to comfort. Questions that are often asked by carers are addressed throughout this chapter.

It is difficult to determine how long each person's journey with dementia will continue. We do know that the end stage of dementia is the inevitable part of the journey that the person, their families and carers must make. How long the end stage of the illness will last is also unknown, but research shows that the remainder of a person's life can usually be measured in months once the end stage of dementia is reached (Mitchell et al., 2009).

How will I know the person has reached the end stage of dementia?

Carers can expect to see significant changes in the following areas as the dementia worsens:

▶ **Cognitive (thinking) ability** – the person will have profound memory loss, which will affect their ability to recognise loved ones or understand basic instructions.

▶ **Speaking ability** – the person will have limited verbal skills and speech may stop altogether.

▶ **Behavioural ability** – the person will no longer be able do things independently (e.g. go to the toilet or wash their hands).

▶ **Functional ability** – the person will be fully dependent on others. Eating and drinking become more difficult, despite being fed by someone.

People die not from the dementia itself, but rather from complications that result as the condition continues to damage the brain. As the person becomes less able to move, eat and drink, they become more susceptible to infections in the lungs (pneumonia) and of the skin (pressure sores). Because dementia mostly affects people over the age of 80 years, people who have dementia also tend to have another long-term illness such as heart disease, diabetes or cancer (Australian Department of Health and Ageing, 2007). These other conditions may also contribute to the person's decline and eventual death.

When it is no longer possible to cure a disease or prevent a person from dying, carers and health professionals must provide care that supports the comfort of the person. Applying what is called a 'palliative approach' does not mean that all treatment and care will be abandoned. Rather, the objective is to support the person living and dying with a life-threatening condition (World Health Organization, 2011).

The aims of a palliative approach to end stage dementia care are to:
- keep the person comfortable and free of pain
- enhance the quality of life for the person and their family
- minimise suffering for the person
- support the person to die peacefully, neither hastening nor postponing death.

Advance care planning

Caring for someone who is dying brings specific needs and challenges to ensure that even after the person has died, carers can be sure that the person's wishes were upheld and that he or she died with peace and dignity. In order to ensure that the person is able to have a 'good death', planning and open communication between the person, their carers and healthcare team are vital. As much as possible, the planning process should involve the person with dementia whilst they still have the mental capacity to make informed decisions about their future care. The person's wishes can be formalised in a legal document called an 'Advance Care Directive' or 'living will' (Cartwright, n.d.).

Ideally, these conversations about end-of-life treatments should take place before the person is in a healthcare establishment such as a hospital or aged care facility. Some of the treatments that may be discussed are antibiotics, blood transfusions, tube feeding, respirator (life support) and resuscitation. Importantly, the person should still be capable of making an informed decision so that they may give or not give consent to future treatments. Having a discussion early on in the illness reduces the need for unnecessary hospitalisation when the person may be in the dying phase of the illness. Knowing what the person would have wanted may also reduce uncertainty for the carers when the person is no longer able to communicate their wishes. To help with these decisions, the treating doctor is responsible for providing information about the overall prognosis; what the benefits and risks of treatments are; the chance of success if the treatment is given; and the effect on the person's quality of life (Kass–Bartelmes & Hughes, 2004).

Advance care planning is about preparing for the future care of the person as, sadly the person with dementia will lose the capacity to make his or her own decisions as the illness progresses. Communicating one's preferences allows the person with a known chronic condition, such as dementia, the opportunity to maintain some control over their future. It is wise to revisit the Advanced Care Plan regularly as decisions made in advance, in a hypothetical situation, may change when the person and their family are faced with the real-life situation.

How do we know someone is dying?

As a carer, you need to know when the dying process is beginning. Research has shown that if carers are aware of the natural complications of end stage dementia, the person may be spared unnecessary, invasive and burdensome treatments in the last weeks or days of life. These treatments may be uncomfortable for the dying person and may prolong their suffering (Mitchell et al., 2009). For carers, coming to this realisation may bring up a range of emotions, such as sadness and perhaps some anxiety, at what may lie ahead. Talking about and planning for the dying process should take place with the appropriate healthcare professionals and with relevant family members.

Carers may begin to notice some significant changes in the person's condition when the dying process has begun. Carers are encouraged to discuss these concerns with the treating doctor who may determine that the dying process has begun when *at least two* of the following four behaviours begin to occur:

- ▸ the person is increasingly sleepy or unconscious
- ▸ the person is in bed all of the time
- ▸ the person is only able to take sips of fluids
- ▸ the person is unable to take tablets.

Caring for the person dying with end stage dementia

As brain function continues to fail in dementia, medical problems begin to increase and treating these problems becomes more and more difficult. Eating and swallowing problems, weight loss, fevers and infections become more frequent and eventually complications from these medical problems will lead to death. Researchers have found that rates of death were high within six months following the development of these problems (Mitchell et al., 2009).

The next part of this chapter will explore the symptoms of end stage dementia, how to recognise them, why they are happening and what carers (and health professionals) can do to help provide comfort to the person.

Symptoms of end stage dementia

Difficulty eating and drinking

How can I recognise it?

As a carer of someone with dementia, you may have already been helping the person eat and drink in the earlier stages of the illness to ensure they were getting enough nutrition and hydration. As the dementia gets worse, despite the food being mashed or pureed and the drinks being thickened, the person may still be eating and drinking less. In the end stages of dementia, the person may not chew their food at all or may hold it in their mouth for a long period of time without swallowing. Food may also simply fall out of the person's mouth because they show a disinterest in food and drink or have an inability to swallow. Carers may worry that the person will 'starve to death' or dehydrate.

Why is it happening?

Signals that come from the brain help to control thoughts about food and coordinate the actions involved in feeding one's self. The confusion caused by dementia affects the co-ordination of all the muscles, including the hands and mouth, making eating and drinking difficult. Eventually, the person is unable to chew food or drink water because of the deterioration of the brain's function caused by dementia. Despite much encouragement from the carer, the person may not be able to eat or drink. This can be frustrating and worrying for the carer; however, when this occurs it is a sign that the person's body is 'winding down' and food and fluids are becoming less important, indicating that the end of life is near.

What can be done to provide comfort?

To watch a person lose the ability to eat food and drink fluids can be very upsetting for carers. Understand that the person's nutritional needs are less and try to feed the person small amounts while they are still willing and able to eat. Avoid trying to force them to eat, as this will increase discomfort and could lead to choking and chest infections. Carers may be worried about dehydration and this is an understandable concern. Dehydration can cause severe dry mouth, agitation and constipation. If these complications from dehydration occur, the doctor may order a slow fluid drip given via a needle under the skin. However, fluids are not appropriate in all cases and should only be given if the person is showing discomfort from dehydration, as described above. There is a risk that the fluid from the drip can accumulate under the skin (because it is not being absorbed properly) or the fluid can accumulate in the lungs, causing breathing to become moist (see the section 'Noisy breathing' on page 173). The sensation of thirst mostly comes from having a dry mouth, so keeping the mouth moist will provide comfort and lessen the feeling of dehydration (see the section 'Dry mouth' on page 170).

Difficulty swallowing (also known as dysphagia)

How can I recognise it?

Swallowing problems are common and are recognised as a sign of end stage dementia. Signs of swallowing problems are coughing or choking whilst the person is eating or drinking.

Why is it happening?

Due to muscle weakness and/or poor coordination, the muscles do not fully close off the airway during the action of swallowing. This can lead to food and fluid entering the lungs (aspiration) and not the stomach; carers will notice this by the cough reflex that is triggered. Repeated bouts of aspiration can cause a severe infection in the lungs, known as aspiration pneumonia.

What can be done to provide comfort?

A speech therapist can assess the person and advise regarding texture of food and positioning during feeding. They can also give information about the severity of the swallowing problem and the risk of aspiration. As swallowing difficulties increase, there are some important considerations that must be made regarding feeding someone who is at the end stage of dementia.

Artificial feeding in end stage dementia

When the person with end stage dementia begins to have trouble swallowing, some medical advice may include the option of inserting a feeding tube into the person's stomach to provide nourishment and hydration. Deciding whether or not to artificially feed a person who is unable to swallow is a complex and highly emotional decision for carers to make.

As discussed earlier, these important decisions can be discussed when an Advanced Care Directive is written. This way the wishes of the person with dementia are known. The person's own preferences for treatment, such as whether to use artificial feeding, guide the carers when the time comes where the person is unable to speak for themselves.

As human beings, we understand that food is essential for life. What is not so well understood is that when a person is in the end stage of a terminal illness, forcing nutrition will not make the person live longer (Candy, Sampson & Jones, 2009; Gillick & Volandes, 2008; Mitchell et al., 2009). In end stage dementia, the body cannot actually process the food. The natural process of dying involves eating less, drinking less and sleeping more. If the decision is made to start artificial feeding via a feeding tube, the person still remains at risk of aspiration pneumonia. This is because even though the food goes from a tube directly into the stomach, reflux can occur and food can still go into the lungs and cause an infection.

Despite artificial feeding, the dying process will continue. It is at that point that the decision to stop the feeds can be more difficult than the decision to start the feeds in the first place. It is important to have an open discussion between the healthcare team and the person's family. The dying process is happening because of the underlying dementia. There comes a time where the body cannot absorb the food because of the dying process.

The person with end stage dementia is not dying because they are not eating and drinking. Rather, they are not eating or drinking *because* they are dying (Therapeutic Guidelines, 2010).

Weight loss

How can I recognise it?
During the end stage of dementia, carers will notice the visual signs of weight loss. Weight loss might be particularly noticeable in the person's face, arms and legs. Bones will be more visible in these areas, as well as around the shoulders and the ribs, and skin may be loose where the body fat once was. Carers will also notice that muscle tone will be greatly reduced, particularly in the arms and legs. Body movement will become less free and the person will need total help to move about. The person may look as though they are in pain, particularly on movement, and they might report feeling cold a lot of the time.

Why is it happening?

Some weight loss may have already occurred earlier in the illness because the person was too confused and did not recognise the food, or they were too restless to eat enough food to maintain their weight.

Complex changes are happening in the person's body during the dying process. The body's metabolism speeds up and where the metabolism once helped build tissues and organs, it is now doing the reverse. The amount of energy gained by nutrition cannot help to slow or stop this natural process. Wasting of the body's muscles and fat is a clear sign that the process of dying is taking place. Weight loss also occurs in the end stages of other diseases such as cancer and heart or liver disease. This kind of severe weight loss cannot be reversed and does not respond to supplements or fortified food or fluids. The person may feel the cold more because they have lost the fat that helps insulate the body and keeps it warm.

What can be done to provide comfort?

Whilst the person is probably spending most or all of the time in bed, moving the limbs carefully and providing some gentle massage with cream or oils can help soothe the body's aches or stiffness. Adequate clothing and warm blankets can also help the person feel warm and comfortable.

Infection and fever

How can I recognise it?

People with end stage dementia are highly susceptible to infections of the lungs (pneumonia) and/or bladder, kidney or urinary tract infections (UTIs). Pneumonia and UTIs can spread to the bloodstream (sepsis) and can cause death in people with end stage dementia. Carers may notice a fever and the signs and symptoms of these types of infections. For example, for pneumonia, coughing may be present, and for a UTI, there may be pain when passing urine.

Why is it happening?

A person in the late stages of dementia will be susceptible to infections because he or she is bedridden, eats and drinks very little and has low immunity to fight off infection. If the person is also having difficulty swallowing, it is highly possible that they may develop aspiration pneumonia. Treating such an infection will depend on the person's wishes, if previously known (e.g. if they have an Advance Care Directive). In the end stage of the disease, difficult choices have to be made. The time comes where the treatment of infection becomes a burden to the dying person. The side effects of the treatments, such as painful injections and diarrhoea from antibiotics, far outweigh the benefits. The alternative to trying to cure the infection is to maintain the person's comfort and allow 'nature to take its course'.

What can be done to provide comfort?

At certain points earlier on the dementia journey, sending a person to hospital when they have a sudden flare up of symptoms, such as an infection or other reversible condition related to the dementia, is generally seen as the appropriate medical treatment. However, once it is established that the person has end stage dementia, the goals of care need to be clear.

Discussions to shift the focus from cure to comfort care should take place between the carer and the medical and nursing staff, with reference to an Advance Care Directive, if one has been made. The carer and healthcare teams should ensure that it is the person with end stage dementia who is at the centre of the discussion and whose needs are being met first and foremost.

Once the decision has been made to stop aggressive or 'active' treatment of infections, pain medication and sedatives can be given as required to control fever, difficulty breathing and pain. Oxygen therapy can also be used if breathing difficulties are as a result of low oxygen levels.

Pressure sores (bed sores)

How can I recognise it?

As the person with dementia becomes less mobile, carers may notice the skin on areas such as the tailbone, heels, outer ankles, elbows and ears might begin to look pink or red. More advanced pressure sores will have black plaques on them. When pressure sores are infected, they may have an unpleasant odour and green or yellow discharge coming from them. Pressure sores can be very painful and in end stage dementia they will not heal well.

Why is it happening?

Pressure sores occur when a bony point in the body is pressed against a surface for an extended period of time. The small blood vessels in the layers of the skin called the epidermis and the dermis get compressed by the bony point and blood that carries oxygen does not get to that area of the skin. The skin cells then die and a wound begins to form.

What can be done to provide comfort?

Prevention of pressure sores is better than cure. Ensure that the person's position is changed approximately every two to four hours. If the person lives in a care facility, the nurses are usually responsible for providing the regular pressure area care, but carers should feel free to assist with this.

Usually, two carers are needed to assist in making these position changes because the person is unable to move themselves in bed. To prevent the bones in the knees and ankles pressing against one another while the person is lying on their side, place a pillow between the lower legs. Pillows can also be used to support the hands and arms.

Carers can also be involved by providing massage to the areas prone to sores (see Figure 14.1). Australian medical sheepskins (not synthetic fibres) are recommended to help protect pressure areas (Palliative Care Australia, 2006). Electric hospital beds with pressure relieving air mattresses can also be hired in care facilities or delivered to the home to help prevent pressure sores.

Once a pressure area develops, healing can be difficult due to deficiencies in nutrition, circulation and immunity related to the end stages of dementia. The main aim of applying dressings to the pressure sore will be to provide comfort. That is, to absorb any discharge, control the odour but not necessarily to heal the wound. Medication can also be given to help relieve the pain from the wound.

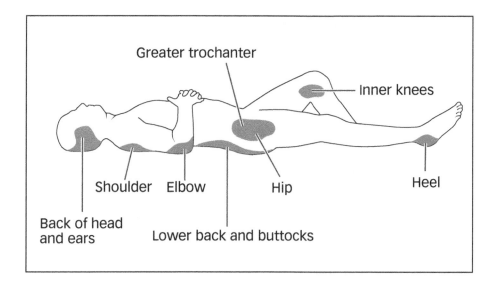

Figure 14.1 Parts of the body that can be affected by pressure, leading to wounds known as 'bed sores' or pressure sores

Pain

How can I recognise it?

As people who are actively dying cannot usually respond in words, it is important to recognise the non-verbal signs of pain. These signs include:

▶ facial grimacing or furrowing of the brow

▶ writhing or constant shifting in bed

▶ moaning or groaning

▶ restlessness and agitation

▶ guarding the area of pain or withdrawing from touch to that area.

Why is it happening?

Pain in dementia has been discussed in detail in Chapter 8. During the dying process, pain can be related to muscle and joint stiffness and inflammation from infection or pressure sores. Pain may also be related to other illnesses the person may have such as heart disease, diabetes or cancer.

What can be done to provide comfort?

Massage and gentle touch can be soothing to a dying person who is experiencing pain. Even though the person may not be able to speak, they can feel your comforting touch. Gentle music can be played and may be comforting to the dying person and to those people sitting with the person. Alternating the person's position left to right every two to four hours can help relieve the pain from being in the one position for too long. Cold or warm packs may also be used to relieve pain.

Mild pain relievers such as paracetamol can help to control aching pain from the bones, skin, muscles and ligaments. It can also provide comfort if there is fever because of an infection. When swallowing becomes difficult, paracetamol suppositories can be given into the rectum (back passage).

Strong pain relievers called opioids (such as morphine, fentanyl and oxycodone) provide the best relief for moderate to severe pain. These medicines are not dangerous when prescribed correctly. Their effects are predictable and doses can be altered easily to manage an individual's pain (Therapeutic Guidelines, 2010).

When the person becomes completely unable to swallow medications, pain relief can be given by an injection under the skin. Medications, such as morphine, can be given on an 'as required' basis if the person is showing signs of discomfort. If more than three doses are required in one day, the doctor should consider giving some medication regularly (Palliative Care Australia, 2006), such as every four hours or via a patch on the skin.

Dry mouth

How can I recognise it?

Carers will notice the person's lips, tongue and inside cheeks look dry and dark pink or red in colour. The tongue in particular may look larger or smaller than usual and may have a shiny or dry appearance.

Why is it happening?

Dry mouth is a very common side effect of some of the medications that may be given to manage pain, agitation or noisy breathing at the end of life. Another common reason for dry mouth is open mouth breathing, which is almost always happening in the unconscious dying person.

What can be done to provide comfort?

A dry mouth will make the person feel thirsty. Frequent small sips of water can be taken if the person can swallow without coughing. In order to keep the person's mouth clean and moist, mouthwash can be used every four hours, but avoid mouthwashes that contain alcohol, which can be even more drying. You can also use plain water with added sodium bicarbonate (baking soda) to cleanse the mouth every four hours or to moisten the mouth in between times. In the last days or hours of life, water can be placed on a swab and gently used to moisten the lips, tongue and inside cheeks. Artificial saliva products are also available. Atomisers (spray bottles) that can be refilled with water can be used to spray a mist into the mouth and can be used every two hours or as required.

Constipation

How can I recognise it?

The first obvious sign of constipation is that the person has not had a bowel motion for at least three days or if they are having difficulty passing a stool. Other signs of constipation can be stomach (abdominal) pains, bloating, nausea or vomiting. The person could also have problems passing urine because of the constipation. Relatively severe constipation can cause the person to have liquid stool. This is called 'overflow' and means that the firmer stool remains in the bowel whilst fluid passes down around it.

Why is it happening?

Constipation occurs when there is a build up of stool (faeces) in the intestine (bowel) and is a common symptom reported in the last stage of life. Generally, a person should have their 'bowels open' or 'pass a motion' each day but at the end of life, once every third day is preferable to keep the person comfortable, particularly if their dietary intake is very low. If their dietary intake is nothing at all (as is found in the last days of life) constipation can still occur in the dying person. The body still makes waste, even if the person does not eat or drink so the person must be observed for signs of discomfort.

People with end stage dementia are at risk of developing constipation for a few reasons including:

▶ inadequate diet and fluids
▶ very little activity and movement
▶ muscle weakness and less awareness of needing to open the bowels
▶ as a side effect of pain medications (opioids).

What can be done to provide comfort?

When the person is no longer able to swallow, rectal suppositories or enemas can be given to stimulate the bowels to open. Towards the last days of life, however, rectal interventions may be inappropriate if the person looks comfortable and is not showing signs of discomfort related to constipation.

Agitation or restlessness

How can I recognise it?

In the last days or weeks of life, carers may notice the person tossing, turning, fidgeting or attempting to get out of bed. The person may also moan or call out. Carers may find it difficult to console the person in this restless or agitated state.

Why is it happening?

The person may have 'all over' pain, or be lying on painful pressure sores, and because they cannot communicate verbally the discomfort is expressed in restlessness. The person may also appear anxious or frightened or may have emotional or spiritual matters left unfinished. Another common source of agitation at the end of life is a full bladder because the person is unable to pass urine. Likewise, constipation may also make the person feel uncomfortable and restless. As the body systems shut down, less oxygen reaches the organs, the metabolism becomes unbalanced and toxins can be released causing severe agitation.

What can be done to provide comfort?

The medical and nursing teams caring for the person should make sure that any reversible causes of agitation are treated. This can include inserting a catheter into the bladder to release the urine or giving an enema to allow the bowel motion to be passed. Pain relief should be given if carers and/or staff suspect the person is agitated because they are in pain.

Restlessness caused by spiritual or emotional pain, fear or anxiety can be eased by reassuring words and touch. If the person is so inclined, a visit from a religious person may help ease emotional unrest. Medications can also be given to help the person settle and sleep, providing a release from these conscious concerns.

Medications, such as sedatives, can be given in liquid form, as a tablet under the tongue or as injections under the skin on an 'as required' basis. Pain relievers and sedation can be given at the same time to keep the person's pain under control and to keep the person settled and asleep. This peaceful, sleepy state allows the person's body to 'wind down' naturally, in comfort and with dignity. The person will be unable to communicate or take food or fluids when they are sedated.

Noisy (rattly) breathing

How can I recognise it?

As the person breathes in and out, carers may begin to hear crackles, bubbling sounds or rattly noises (this is sometimes called the 'death rattle'). This will usually be noticed when the person is in the last days or hours of life. The sound of noisy breathing can be very distressing for carers and onlookers, some of whom may worry that the person could suffocate or choke.

Why is it happening?

Fluid (including saliva) or phlegm builds up in the throat, windpipe and/or the lungs. This can be as a result of aspiration (taking food or fluid into the lungs instead of the stomach), aspiration pneumonia (chest infection from aspiration) or from fluid shifting into incorrect places around the organs. If the person is too weak to cough up and clear it, the congestion remains there and can be heard rattling with each breath in and out. Rattly breathing does not necessarily mean that the person is finding it hard to breathe (see the section 'Breathing difficulties and changes in breathing patterns').

What can be done to provide comfort?

Generally, when noisy breathing occurs the person is in an unconscious state, so often they are not aware of any discomfort. However, if the person is restless and seems in discomfort, positioning the head and chest in a 45-degree angle and/or positioning the person onto their side can help relieve congestion. Medications can also be used to dry up the congestion and these are generally given as an injection under the skin. Sedative medication can also be useful to keep the person in a deep sleep so they are not aware of any discomfort because of noisy breathing. If the sound can still be heard but the breathing remains regular, and the person's facial expressions look calm, this is a sure sign the person is not uncomfortable because of the noisy breathing.

Breathing difficulties and changes in breathing patterns

How can I recognise it?

As the last days or hours of life approach, carers will notice that breathing appears difficult for the person; this is often called 'laboured breathing'. Breathing may also become shallow, fast and irregular in pattern. Just before the time when the last breaths are taken, carers may notice that the breathing rate slows and long gaps are taken between breaths; some gasping of breath may also occur. Breaths will then eventually fade and stop. After the breaths appear to have stopped, an occasional breath or action of the jaw may be noticed. These last movements will also stop after a brief period of time (up to a few minutes).

Why is it happening?

Laboured breathing occurs because the lungs are no longer able to work efficiently to deliver oxygen to the body. The lungs have to work harder to perform this task, which is vital to life in the human body. The irregular patterns are a normal part of the dying process as all the body systems are shutting down.

What can be done to provide comfort?

These changes in the breathing are a normal part of the dying process and the person experiencing them is usually unaware as they are unconscious. If breathing is laboured and the person looks uncomfortable (e.g. they are shifting in the bed and looking restless), morphine can be useful to reduce the feeling of breathlessness. Other medications, such as sedatives, can also relax breathing and will make the person sleep and keep them settled.

Placing a gentle fan on or opening a window can help reduce the feeling of being closed in, while positioning the person's head and upper body at a 45-degree angle can also help laboured breathing.

Frequently asked questions

Frequently asked questions about morphine at the end of life

The doctor seems reluctant to prescribe morphine. Why is this?

Whether we like it or not, morphine and other opioids have a stigma attached to them. High doses given to people who have not had opioids before can cause breathing to slow right down or even stop. Therefore, if not experienced in prescribing – starting from a small dose and gradually building upwards – some doctors may lack the confidence and not know at which dose it is safe to begin. Nurses in residential aged care facilities can also have similar fears and worries about giving morphine, even if the doctor has prescribed it.

How much morphine can the person have? Will they become addicted?

Each person's pain medication needs are different. There is no maximum dose of morphine and when used to provide relief from pain, people will not develop an addiction. Opioid drugs, such as morphine, are addictive when abused by people with no physical pain (i.e for recreation) who then develop an emotional dependency on them. Once a person with physical pain has been on morphine for a while, tolerance to the medication can develop and the dose may need to be increased slightly.

Is the morphine causing the person to be sleepy all the time?

In the first few days, taking morphine can make the person drowsy but this subsides fairly quickly. Generally, a person with end stage dementia will be sleeping more often because of the disease, not just because of the medication.

I knew of someone who was started on morphine 'at the end' and they died soon after. Will morphine make the person die more quickly?

This is a common story and, sadly, is a result of the myth that morphine is what causes people to die. One reason that this myth is perpetuated is that people (including some doctors, nurses and carers alike) feel that they should keep morphine 'in reserve' for when the pain is severe, using morphine only as a last resort (Notcutt & Gibbs, 2010). This practice is partly fuelled by fear around the drug because of its perceived potency and side effects. Compounding this further, unrealistic fears around addiction delay the acceptance of using the drug as a pain reliever for moderate to strong pain.

So by the time doctors come around to prescribing, nurses come around to giving and carers come around to accepting morphine to relieve pain, the person has come quite near to the time death was already likely to occur. The fact that the morphine was given (eventually) and the person died is a pure coincidence of timing.

Frequently asked questions about dying

Can he/she still hear us even though they are unconscious?

It is widely believed that when a person is dying, 'hearing is the last sense to go'. It is helpful for both the dying person and for the carer that you continue to speak to the person even when they cannot speak back. This may be a time where you may wish to say things that were previously not said. It may also be a time to say goodbye. If you find yourself talking to a person who cannot communicate back, you may want to just let them know you are there and hold their hand. Despite being unconscious, the person can still feel your touch and this can be very reassuring.

How long before the person dies?

It is impossible to predict just when a person will die, even if the person has been 'actively dying' for hours or days. Some experienced staff members may be able to recognise physical signs that death may be close and advise you on when to call other relatives or when to stay overnight. However, even those who keep a constant vigil by the bedside need to leave occasionally to go to the bathroom or to get a drink and risk not being with the person right at the moment of death. At this stage, when death is likely to be very near, ensure that you have not left anything unsaid, just in case you are not there right at the moment of their last breath. It is true that some carers who have 'missed the moment' are reassured that perhaps the dying person chose a moment when they were alone to peacefully slip away.

What are some signs we can look for to know death may be close?

Carers will notice changes in breathing, as mentioned earlier in the section 'Breathing difficulties and changes in breathing patterns'. Gaps between breaths usually means that death is only hours or even minutes away. The colour in the person's face will look paler and may have a slightly yellow tone. As the body's circulation closes down, to be closer to the major organs blood is drawn away from the extremities. The hands and feet may, therefore, feel cool and skin may appear mottled and blue or purple in colour. The person is usually comfortable and not aware of these temperature changes.

How will I know the person has died?

Even though the person's death is expected, you may still experience some shock when the moment actually arrives. This may be because you have been busy comforting family members, dealing with enquiries about the person or talking to staff. The final moment of death will no doubt conjure up many emotions. There is no right or wrong way to feel or react – do what feels right for you at the time.

Some physical signs you may notice when the person has died include the following:

▶ they will not be breathing
▶ they will have no pulse
▶ they will be totally unresponsive
▶ their skin will begin to cool fairly quickly
▶ their eyes may remain open or be closed
▶ their jaw will be relaxed and the mouth may be open
▶ their body may relax and air or fluid may be released.

Who do I call when the person has died?

There is no urgency or rush once the person has died. For some carers, the period immediately after death can be a precious time to sit with the person and reflect. For others, this may be a time to leave the room and take a break. Once again, do what feels right for you at the time. Grief is a very individual emotion and each person deals with the dying process in their own way.

If you are in a hospital or aged care facility, you may want to let the nursing staff know that the person has died so they can offer advice and support. If the person dies at home expectedly, you *do not* need to call an ambulance. You will, however, need to contact the family doctor to come to the home and certify that the person has died. Organising a doctor ahead of time is a good idea as there is a good chance the person's death may fall out of working hours. You should also be aware of your local after hours service numbers to assist with this process. If the person dies overnight, they may stay in the home until the morning, so you may leave calling the doctor until then.

After the doctor has certified that the person has died, he or she will provide you with a medical certificate of death or an interim certificate to confirm that the person has died. You may then call the funeral director who will come to collect the person's body from the home.

After the person has died

The role of caring for a person with dementia becomes a huge part of a carer's life. When the person has died, a sense of loss can be felt on many levels. For many, loss has already occurred as the person with dementia has lost their ability to recognise loved ones and to care for themselves. Although the death was likely to have been expected, carers may experience a range of thoughts and feelings in the days, weeks, months and years after the death. Grief is very individual and carers should do what feels right and is comfortable at the time. In the hours following the death, carers may feel numb or in shock. As time passes, carers may feel that they cannot stop thinking about the person or may find it hard to accept that they have really died. The carer may think that they can hear or see the person, or that the deceased will arrive home again. For many, a sense of relief is felt that the person is no longer suffering. While relief is understandable, and indeed expected, it may also stir up the emotion of guilt for feeling this way. A wide range of emotions may be felt including anger, depression and exhaustion. These feelings are normal and should be acknowledged and not ignored.

Carers should understand that grief is an ongoing process and there may be times of upset months or even years after the death of the person. It is vital that carers consider their own physical and mental health during the process of grieving. It is important to keep in contact with friends and family and remember that talking about one's emotions may prevent the build up of tension and depressive feelings. If the carer feels physically sick or depressed, it is advisable to see the family doctor. Talking about one's feelings to a professional, a trusted friend or relative or in a support group setting is an important step in grieving a loss and carrying on with life in a healthy way.

Working through grief and adapting to a significant loss involves time and an understanding that there will be good days and not-so-good days. It was once thought that detaching oneself from the lost person was the way to adapt to a loss. Now experts believe that mourners can adapt to the loss by maintaining an emotional connection to the lost person whilst carrying on with life (Worden, 2009). This may take the form of memorialising the person in some way such as having an object close that belonged to the person that died or undertaking a project to honour the person's life. Again, individuals should do what feels right for them.

Conclusion

Even though dementia cannot be cured, carers and their supporting healthcare teams aim to provide the person with the best quality of life possible. As the journey with dementia comes to an end, care is focused on the comfort of the person rather than trying to cure conditions related to the dementia. Some carers may be presented with difficult decisions along the way; however, it is hoped that reading this chapter has enabled some important conversations to take place before the end of the journey is reached. Sadly, dementia will shorten a person's life; however, death should be respected as a natural part of life. Understanding the dying process may better equip carers for what is perhaps the most difficult part of the journey alongside the person with dementia.

References

Australian Department of Health and Ageing. (2007). *Dementia and physical co-morbidity — Facilitator's guide.* Retrieved from http://www.rhef.com.au/wp-content/uploads/616b_facil_lr.pdf

Candy, B., Sampson, E. L., & Jones, L. (2009). Enteral tube feeding in older people with advanced dementia: Findings from a Cochrane systematic review. *International Journal of Palliative Nursing, 15*(8), 396–404.

Cartwright, C. (n.d.). *Advance health care directive.* Coffs Harbour, NSW: Aged Services Learning and Research Collaboration, Southern Cross University. Retrieved from http://ntwebhost2.pacific.net.au/~cotaweb/docs/AdvanceHealthCareDirective.pdf

Gillick, M. R., & Volandes, A. E. (2008). The standard of caring: Why do we still use feeding tubes in patients with advanced dementia? *Journal of the American Medical Directors Association, 9*(5), 364–367. doi: 10.1016/j.jamda.2008.03.011

Kass-Bartelemes, B. L., & Hughes, R. G. (2004). Advance care planning: Preferences for care at the end of life. *Journal of Pain & Palliative Care Pharmacotherapy, 18*(1), 87–109.

Mitchell, S. L., Teno, J. M., Kiely, D. K., Shaffer, M. L., Jones, R. N., Prigerson, H. G., Volicer, L., Givens, J. L., & Hamel, M. B. (2009). The clinical course of advanced dementia. *New England Journal of Medicine, 361*(16), 1529–1538.

Notcutt, W., & Gibbs, G. (2010). Inadequate pain management: Myth, stigma and professional fear. *Postgraduate Medical Journal, 86,* 453–458. doi:10.1136/pgmj.2008.077677

Palliative Care Australia. (2006). *Guidelines for palliative approach in residential aged care* (Enhanced edition). Retrieved from http://www.palliativecare.org.au/Portals/46/Aged%20Care/The%20Guidelines%202006.pdf

Therapeutic Guidelines. (2010). *Therapeutic guidelines: Palliative care (Version 3).* Melbourne: Therapeutic Guidelines Limited.

Worden, J. M. (2009). *Grief counseling and grief therapy: A Handbook for the mental health practitioner* (4th ed.). New York: Springer Publishing Company.

World Health Organization. (2011). *WHO definition of palliative care* [webpage]. Retrieved from http://www.who.int/cancer/palliative/definition/en/

Chapter 15

THE EXPERIENCE
OF CARING

Jane Thompson
Australian National University

Chapter outcomes

When you have completed this chapter you will be able to:

▸ appreciate the personal experience of dementia caring

▸ understand how being a carer of a person with dementia affects the carer's health

▸ recognise the factors influencing the carer's ability to cope.

Keywords

dementia, carers' health, depression, anxiety, caregiver burden

---

Introduction

Dementia caregiving is hard. It is complicated and often unpredictable. For many carers – and here (and in the following chapter) I am referring to those individuals who provide ongoing, generally unpaid, non-professional or informal care for a family member, relative or friend – it may be the most challenging circumstance in which they find themselves in their lifetime. It is difficult in part because many of the ordinary, day-to-day decisions that have to be made by carers of people with dementia are fundamentally ethical (Hughes, 2010). Carers are often asking 'What is the right thing to do?' or 'Am I doing the wrong thing?' While the motivations to take on the role of carer may vary (a sense of love or reciprocity, spiritual fulfilment, a sense of duty, guilt, social pressures or, in rare instances, greed), most probably feel they don't really have a choice. Carers who are still of working age may have different attitudes to and expectations of their role than, for example, older carers who have enjoyed many years with their spouse and embrace their caring role as the final chapter in their lives. Nonetheless, most are likely to feel ill-prepared for the long journey. It is not a journey that can be undertaken alone. It generally involves a constant cycle of adjustment, followed by crisis requiring adaptation and then a further adjustment phase – this is repeated over and over. Carers will inevitably have to draw on all their own strengths and inner resources and will need to access and accept help from many others along the way. The old adage 'It takes a village to raise a child', rephrased in the dementia context, applies: 'It takes a village to care for a person with dementia'.

For me, caring for my husband through his rapid journey with the most common form of the progressive dementias, Alzheimer's disease, was certainly the most heart wrenching, agonising and painful experience I had ever confronted. This wasn't part of our marriage contract! I thought, 'This couldn't be happening to us'. My husband was 68 at the time of his diagnosis. He had been fit, healthy, even youthful, ever since I had known him. He had a distinguished career as a scientist, an endlessly inquiring mind and fascination with the world around him. He adored me. We had plans for our future together (even though he was 14 years older than me). It was a future with relative freedom from responsibilities as our sons had gained independence, which meant we could travel and share more time together doing some of the things that had necessarily been deferred. But here I was, in dark and unfamiliar territory. I cannot describe this experience any more eloquently than Joyce Carol Oates does in her book *A Widow's Story* (Oates, 2011), which she wrote after her husband's sudden unexpected death. She writes about meeting an old friend Rachael whose husband has been afflicted with early-onset Alzheimer's. Oates poignantly describes her as being in the 'cruel twilit state of being *not-yet-a-widow*' and writes:

> *Terrible as losing a husband is, there is perhaps a worse predicament in losing the person he was; living with him on a daily basis as he deteriorates; feeling you have no choice finally, as Rachael felt, but to arrange for him to be hospitalized ... Rachael is very thin, her skin is very pale, she too is one of the walking wounded (2011, p. 326).*

Oates contemplates who has been less lucky: the wife who loses her husband suddenly or the one who loses him by 'slow excruciating degrees'. Oates would like to comfort Rachael: 'You've had a trauma. You must take care of yourself.' This is salient advice. Just as flight passengers are instructed to fit their own oxygen masks first before trying to help others, so too, attending to and maintaining one's own health – physical, mental and spiritual – is essential to being able to care for another's. Taking personal control over one's health is an often espoused principle. However, taking such control may seem impossible for a carer who may be feeling distinctly lacking in control over their life, overwhelmed and not confident that they have the appropriate skills and energy to do this. Perhaps it might be more helpful to say to them: 'You must take care of yourself and you will need some help to do that.'

Every dementia carer's journey will be unique. Challenges will vary for spousal carers, those caring for a parent, carers of an older partner or one with younger onset dementia. In addition, same-sex partners, persons from varied cultural backgrounds, races or ethnicities will all encounter special challenges. However, while each journey is unique, there will also be some commonalities between them. For most the experience will mean facing the pain of truly losing someone they love and most will feel ill-prepared and ill-equipped to take on the caring role before them. There is no road map, no one-size-fits-all manual; each will need to write their own and set then reset their own compass.

It is important not to be fooled about the reality of caring for someone with dementia. I found realistic depictions most helpful. These included the book *Elegy for Iris* and the motion picture *Iris* based on the true story of Iris Murdoch's battle with Alzheimer's disease, as told by her husband John Bayley. This resonated with my experience, as did the very poignant, though gruelling to watch, movie *A Song for Martin*. I didn't want the sanitised version of how things might be. No images of loving couples enjoying their twilight years, smiling while strolling hand in hand along golden sandy beaches with nauseatingly romantic messages about enjoying what you have left together. No, I wanted affirmation of my experience; that this was agony for both the carer and the person with dementia. My husband was fraught with frustration and anxiety and was clearly in great emotional pain. 'Please help me, I'm afraid' was his mantra. I felt helpless but to say 'I'm here; I'll help you.' It was absolute agony watching someone I loved, with whom I had a past but now no future, struggling to make sense of a world that was shrinking and becoming a frightening and alienating place in which he couldn't work out where he belonged any more. I remember his poignant plea 'I don't know who I am any more.' Looking at me and asking 'Where is Jane, my wife?' Looking at our children and asking painfully 'Is he one of ours?' What was I to do when, in frustration, he would beat his head with closed fists or bang his head against the brick walls until he injured himself, sheer frustration at not knowing how to perform simple tasks any more. While strategies I learnt to use to control these behavioural and psychological symptoms worked to some extent, ultimately only antipsychotic medication could calm him. Should I have felt guilty for failing and resorting to potentially harmful medications? No – I did the best I could under the circumstances. I was a 'good enough' carer and perhaps this is all we can do.

This chapter summarises the research that has investigated the impact of caring for a person with dementia on the carer. There are two essential messages: firstly, that being the carer of a person with dementia is hard on the carer; and secondly, that given how important the role is, looking after the carer is vital as it enables the carer to provide better care.

The health of carers

Caring for a person with dementia exacts a significant toll on the carer's health and wellbeing (Brodaty & Donkin, 2009; Dupuis, Epp & Smale, 2004). Dementia caring may be associated with a higher level of stress than caring for someone with functional impairment from another type of chronic illness (Pinquart & Sorensen, 2007). Alzheimer's and other dementias are progressive and disabling often requiring an intensive level of care. Along with the inevitable decline in memory and physical functioning, the person being cared for is likely to exhibit challenging behavioural and psychological symptoms. Carers may feel ill-equipped or unable to help with these distressing features of the disease. Furthermore, depending on their life stage and relationship with the person they care for, carers will often be balancing caregiving with other demands such as child rearing, career and relationships. They may also experience financial stress both direct (e.g. cost of medications and home modifications) and indirect (e.g. loss of earnings due to relinquishing of paid work).

Physical health

The stresses associated with any caregiving role negatively impact on carers' physical health. Higher caregiving demands, such as that experienced by dementia carers, have a stronger impact. In general, compared with non-caregivers, carers are more likely to have a long-term medical problem (e.g. high blood pressure, heart disease, cancer, diabetes or arthritis); higher levels of stress hormones, insulin and blood clotting factors; spend more days sick with an infectious disease; have a weaker immune response to the influenza vaccine; slower wound healing; higher levels of obesity; and perceive their own health status to be lower (Patterson & Grant, 2003).

In terms of increased risk of death, older people who feel stressed while taking care of their disabled spouses may be more likely to die than carers who are not feeling stressed (Schulz & Beach, 1999). For both men and women, there is an increased likelihood of their own death if their spouse is hospitalised and the risk of death has been found to be highest for spouses whose partner is hospitalised with a diagnosis of dementia (Christakis & Allison, 2006).

One of the reasons carers may have health problems is because they are less likely to take good care of themselves. They may be less likely to get needed medical care, fill a prescription and engage in health preventative behaviours. Compared with the time before taking on the role, they may be less likely to get enough sleep, cook healthy meals and get enough physical activity.

Sleep, or lack thereof, is of particular concern for dementia carers. Sleep disturbances in people with dementia and their carers are highly prevalent and impact significantly on quality of life for both (Lee & Thomas, 2011; McCurry et al., 2009). Dementia carers have been reported to sleep less and to have reduced sleep efficiencies. Sleep disturbances have also been linked to poorer physical health outcomes. Such sleep disturbances, often associated with nocturnal wandering of the care recipient, are cited by many carers as a major reason for seeking the permanent institutionalisation of the person with dementia. Although sleep problems are common in carers they are often not reported and so remain untreated.

Psychological, mental and emotional health

Dementia caring is associated with a high level of burden (Etters, Goodall & Harrison, 2008). Burden encompasses both objective burden (which, in relation to dementia care, reflects the dependency of the person with dementia and the level of behavioural disturbance) and subjective burden or strain (the appraisal of burden by the carer including their evaluation of the physical and emotional impact, their psychological state and resources). Both objective and subjective burden may be higher among dementia carers than non-dementia carers. Not surprisingly, high levels of burden impact significantly on carers' quality of life and carers often report feeling overwhelmed by their caring role and loss of control of their situation.

Depression and/or depressive symptoms are more prevalent in dementia carers than in either non-caregivers or carers of other chronically ill people (Cuijpers 2005; Schoenmakers, Buntinx & Delepeleire, 2010). Frequently, the symptoms only arise after the caring role commences. Depression is more common in women carers than in men and spouses are more likely to experience depression than non-spousal carers. Dementia carers may also suffer from anxiety (Cooper, Balamurali & Livingston, 2007). This encompasses feelings of worry and fear, as well as physical symptoms including muscular tension and other bodily symptoms.

Feelings of loss and grief are also frequent among dementia carers (Frank, 2007). Grief includes both anticipatory grief (a complex concept that encompasses grief in anticipation of the future loss of a loved one, in addition to previously experienced and current losses as a result of the terminal illness) and ambiguous loss (a particular form of grief that centres on the fact that the carer has lost the person they know and love as their personalities, memories and ability to function are overtaken by their dementia; they are still living but they are increasingly gone). Carers can experience prolonged patterns of grieving that begin before the death of the person with dementia. Some may experience complicated grief after the death with symptoms including a sense of disbelief; anger and bitterness; recurrent painful emotions, with intense yearning and longing for the deceased; and a preoccupation with thoughts of the loved one, often including distressing intrusive thoughts related to the death (Schulz et al., 2006). Avoidance of situations and activities that serve as reminders of the painful loss is also common. Complicated grief is more common among carers with high levels of depressive symptoms and burden prior to the person's death, as well as those who report positive features of the care-giving experience; or who have been caring for a more cognitively impaired person.

Dementia carers may also experience social isolation through lack of personal time and opportunities to socialise. Further, because of the stigma of the disease, family and friends may distance themselves (Charlesworth et al., 2011). Without support, carers can feel emotionally and physically burdened. A perception of low emotional support may increase feelings of loneliness. For long-term partners where one is diagnosed with dementia, the other has to face the effective loss of companionship and support of a life partner. Issues relating to sexuality and intimacy are also important.

Caring for someone with dementia, a spouse in particular, can also affect carers' cognitive performance (Vitaliano et al., 2011). Dementia caring results in increased exposure to a range of factors that are associated with an increased risk of cognitive decline. These include psychosocial factors (e.g. less mental stimulation, social isolation, loneliness and depression), behavioural factors (e.g. difficulty maintaining healthy eating habits and physical activity) and physiological factors (e.g. an increase in stress hormones).

The transition of the person with dementia to residential care often occurs because of poor or declining health of the carer and the increasing burden. While providing some relief from the burden of care for the carer, this phase of the journey can also bring stresses. Most carers want to remain closely involved in the lives of the person they have been caring for at home. However, poor family–staff relationships can have a detrimental effect on the health and wellbeing of carers with unmet expectations about care being a source of considerable stress (Haesler, Bauer & Nay, 2010).

Providing care at the end of the life of the person with dementia is also often very demanding for the carer, particularly for those providing in-home care. This is a time when carers experience high levels of depressive symptoms but may show remarkable resilience after the death. When death is preceded by a protracted and stressful period of caregiving, carers often report considerable relief at the death itself – both for themselves and for the patient. Carers' depressive symptoms often subside significantly within a year of the death (Schulz et al., 2003).

Positive aspects of caring: growing and gaining strength from caregiving

While the burdens and stresses experienced by dementia carers have been explored extensively, there has been less research from the strengths perspective focusing on how people might grow stronger or gain from a stressful situation. Expressed gains during the time caring for a relative with dementia include:

▶ positive experiences (e.g. enjoying togetherness, sharing activities and feeling a reciprocal bond)
▶ spiritual growth and increased faith
▶ personal growth (e.g. being more patient and understanding, becoming stronger and more resilient, having increased self-awareness and being more knowledgeable)
▶ gains in relationships (e.g. experiencing an improvement in relationship with the care recipient, with others in the family or in ability to interact with other older people)
▶ feelings of mastery and accomplishment (Netto, Goh & Phillip, 2009; Sanders, 2005).

Carers not expressing gains may be those providing caregiving in isolation, without much assistance from others.

Diverse groups of carers

There is a diversity of caregiving situations that carers find themselves in, in terms of the type of dementia involved, the culture and ethnicity of carers, whether they are in a rural or remote location, as well as their age and sexual orientation. The experiences of such a diverse group of carers will vary considerably and it is a challenge to meet what is likely to be a diverse set of needs.

Much of the research has focused on carers of persons with Alzheimer's disease. However, persons with Lewy body dementia may present a unique set of symptoms and challenges to carers compared with other types of dementia (Leggett et al., 2011). Prominent issues include motor impairment, difficulties with activities of daily living, recurrent behavioural and emotional problems and diagnostic difficulties. These problems are likely to affect carers' subjective burden and there may be significant unmet needs in terms of appropriate support services. Caregiver burden among Alzheimer's disease carers compared with carers of those with vascular dementia (dementia associated with problems of circulation of blood to the brain) has not been found to differ but may be more related to particular symptoms in the care recipient (e.g. psychotic symptoms) (Yeager et al., 2010). There is very little published research on specific issues faced by carers of persons with Pick's disease, which affects the frontal lobes of the brain, but in some cases can affect the temporal lobes.

Issues relating to caring for persons with younger onset dementia have received more attention recently (Svanberg, Spector & Stott, 2011; van Vliet et al., 2010). Younger onset dementia carers are often unprepared for the task and may experience high levels of burden, stress and depression. This may be related to their phase in life; for example, they may still be pursuing a career, have financial commitments and/ or a young family. Getting a diagnosis can be difficult and there may be genetic implications for any children. These carers may also suffer intense feelings of grief, especially as the condition may deteriorate more quickly than in older people. On top of this, appropriate services may not be available and they may feel more isolated.

Little research has been done to assess the impact on children of those diagnosed with younger onset dementia. Studies to date indicate that children may experience high levels of burden but moderate levels of resilience (Svanberg, Stott & Spector, 2010). Adaptation may involve moving through grief to emotional detachment and increased maturity.

One special group with an increased risk of younger onset dementia are people with Down syndrome. The carers of these people face additional challenges in diagnosis, management and other issues and therefore require special attention.

Other groups who may experience additional challenges beyond those directly related to caregiving are same-sex partners of people with dementia (Birch, 2009). Existing interventions and support services may not meet their needs or address the issues they face. They may experience prejudice and insensitivity in their interactions with health services, a lack of social and emotional support and workplace and legal difficulties.

Distress from caregiving may be expressed differently among people of varying ethnic backgrounds (Brodaty & Donkin, 2009). Further, people from ethnic minorities and indigenous groups may be less likely to have access to or to use mental health services. Contributing factors include a lack of understanding about dementia; language or other communication barriers; a lack of general practitioner knowledge of cultural differences in expression of mental illness and distress; a distrust of Western medicine; ethnocentric attitudes; and incorrect assumptions (for instance, that certain ethnic groups will look after their relatives and do not require services).

What features exacerbate or ameliorate the negative effects of caring?

Numerous studies have tried to determine whether any particular characteristics or attitudes of carers might influence the level of psychological distress they experience. Those who are motivated by a sense of duty, guilt or social and cultural norms may be more likely to resent their role and suffer greater psychological distress than carers with more positive motivations. Carers who identify more beneficial components of their role experience less burden, better health and relationships, and greater social support. The strongest predictors of caregiver burden are a sense of 'role captivity' (carer feelings of being trapped in their role); caregiver overload (e.g. fatigue and burnout); adverse life events outside of the caregiving role; and relationship quality (Brodaty & Donkin, 2009).

Spouses who are inexperienced caregivers may be most vulnerable to negative outcomes and, further, spouses who rate their marriage as strong and satisfying may experience less of a burden than spouses who rate their marriage more negatively (Hellstrom, Nolan & Lundh, 2007). 'Finding meaning' may also buffer the burden for carers of spouses with dementia. Personality, for example having a sense of optimism and control, may also be important.

Difficulties may arise when a person with dementia is in a second (or later) marriage, particularly when he or she has children from a previous marriage. There may be disputes about financial, legal or guardianship issues. When people marry close to the time that they begin to develop symptoms of dementia, further issues can arise regarding their capacity to marry and possibly the motivation of their partner to become their carer as there may be less well developed feelings of reciprocity and obligation (Brodaty & Donkin, 2009).

Self-efficacy for managing dementia (that is, the belief that one can perform a specific task or behaviour) may protect against burden and depression in dementia carers (Romero-Moreno et al., 2011). Avoidance and dysfunctional coping strategies may predispose carers to higher levels of distress, whereas successful caregiving seems to be based on the use of problem-oriented strategies early in the disease when solutions are still available. Self-efficacy for controlling upsetting thoughts may be particularly effective for carers who report high burden scores, attenuating the impact of burden on carers' distress (depression and anxiety).

Characteristics of the dementia care recipient may also exacerbate the burden of caregiving. These include, for example, a lack of insight, changes in personality, disruptive behaviours, level of dependence, duration and severity of dementia and their educational level (Garcia-Alberca, Lara & Berthier, 2011).

An understanding of why some carers manage well and others do less well is critical. Differences can be seen both as an individual difference between carers and as a product of the caring situation at a given moment in the carer's journey. More focus is now being placed on designing models of care based on positive concepts of resilience and survivorship, which aim to build on carers' strengths (Eagar et al., 2007).

Practical advice for carers

Some practical advice for carers is listed below. Carers should:
- be aware of the negative consequences of caring for a person with dementia for their own health
- ensure that they attend to their own needs as well as those of the person they care for (dementia caring is hard work!)
- try to maintain physical health through good nutrition, exercise and getting adequate sleep
- remember that they will need emotional support to help with inevitable feelings of grief and loss that accompany the dementia caring journey.

In the words of one carer, Dianne:

> *Without the support of our psychologist reinforcing my rights as an individual, I would be back where I was four years ago; totally ignoring my needs and focusing solely on those of my husband.*

Conclusion

Most dementia carers provide a level of care that negatively impacts on their own health and wellbeing. Dementia carers are 'the often forgotten patient'. Dementia caring is particularly stressful because of the difficulties carers face in managing the behavioural and psychological changes that occur in the person they care for. In addition, carers may be particularly at risk of suffering ill consequences from chronic sleep loss superimposed upon the stress of their caregiving role. An extensive body of research has investigated interventions to maintain or improve carers' health and wellbeing and is explored in the following chapter.

References

Birch, H. (2009). *Dementia, lesbians and gay men.* Alzheimer's Australia Paper 15. Canberra: Alzheimer's Australia.

Brodaty, H., & Donkin M. (2009). Family caregivers of people with dementia. *Dialogues in Clinical Neuroscience, 11*(2), 217–228.

Charlesworth, G. Burnell, K., Beecham, J., Hoare, Z., Hoe, J., Wenborn, J., Knapp, M., Russell, I., Woods, B., & Orrell, M. (2011). Peer support for family carers of people with dementia, alone or in combination with group reminiscence in a factorial design: study protocol for a randomised controlled trial. *Trials,* 12, 205.

Christakis, N. A., & Allison P. D. (2006). Mortality after the hospitalization of a spouse. *New England Journal of Medicine, 354,* 719–730.

Cooper, C., Balamurali, T. B. S., & Livingston, G. (2007). A systematic review of the prevalence and covariates of anxiety in caregivers of people with dementia. *International Psychogeriatrics, 19,* 175–195.

Cuijpers, P. (2005). Depressive disorders in caregivers of dementia patients: A systematic review. *Aging & Mental Health, 9,* 325–330.

Dupuis, S. L., Epp T., & Smale, B. (2004). *Caregivers of persons with dementia: Roles, experiences, supports, and coping. A literature review.* Waterloo, ON: Murray Alzheimer Research and Education Program, University of Waterloo.

Eagar, K., Owen, A., Williams, K., Westera, A., & Marosszeky, N. (2007). *Effective caring: A synthesis of the international evidence on carer needs and interventions.* Wollongong, NSW: Centre for Health Service Development, University of Wollongong.

Etters, L., Goodall, D., & Harrison, B. (2008). Caregiver burden among dementia patient caregivers: A review of the literature. *Journal of the American Academy of Nurse Practitioners, 20,* 423–428.

Frank, J. B. (2007). Evidence for grief as the major barrier faced by Alzheimer caregivers: A qualitative analysis. *American Journal of Alzheimer's Disease & Other Dementias, 22,* 516–527.

Garcia-Alberca, J. M., Lara, J. P., & Berthier, M. L. (2011). Anxiety and depression in caregivers are associated with patient and caregiver characteristics in Alzheimer's disease. *International Journal of Psychiatry in Medicine, 41,* 57–69.

Haesler, E., Bauer, M., & Nay, R. (2010). Recent evidence on the development and maintenance of constructive staff-family relationships in the care of older people – A report on a systematic review update. *International Journal of Evidence-Based Healthcare, 8*(2), 45–74.

Hellstrom, I., Nolan, M., & Lundh, U. (2007). Sustaining 'couplehood' : Spouses' strategies for living positively with dementia. *Dementia, 6*(3), 383–409.

Hughes, J. (2010). *Ethical issues and decision making in dementia care.* Alzheimer's Australia Paper 20. Canberra: Alzheimer's Australia.

Lee, D. R., & Thomas, A. J. (2011). Sleep in dementia and caregiving – assessment and treatment implications: A review. *International Psychogeriatrics, 23*(2), 190–201.

Leggett, A. N., Zarit, S., Taylor, A., & Galvin, J. (2011). Stress and burden among caregivers of patients with Lewy body dementia. *Gerontologist, 51*(1), 76–85.

McCurry, S. M., Gibbons, L. E., Logsdon, R., Vitiello, M., & Teri, L. (2009). Insomnia in caregivers of persons with dementia: Who is at risk and what can be done about it? *Sleep Medicine Clinics, 4,* 519–526.

Netto, N. R., Goh, Y. N. J., & Phillip, Y. L. K. (2009). Growing and gaining through caring for a loved one with dementia. *Dementia, 8*(2), 245–261.

Oates, J. C. (2011). *A widow's story: A memoir.* New York: Ecco Press.

Patterson, T. L., & Grant, I. (2003). Interventions for caregiving in dementia: Physical outcomes. *Current Opinion in Psychiatry, 16,* 629–633.

Pinquart, M., & Sorensen, S. (2007). Correlates of physical health of informal caregivers: A meta-analysis. *Journals of Gerontology, Series B: Psychological Sciences & Social Sciences, 62*(2), 126–137.

Romero-Moreno, R. Losada, A., Mausbach, B. T., Márquez-González, M., Patterson, T. L., & López, J. (2011). Analysis of the moderating effect of self-efficacy domains in different points of the dementia caregiving process. *Aging & Mental Health, 15*(2), 221–231.

Sanders, S. (2005). Is the glass half empty or full? Reflections on strain and gain in caregivers of individuals with Alzheimer's disease. *Social Work in Health Care, 40*(3), 57–73.

Schoenmakers, B., Buntinx, F., & Delepeleire, J. (2010). Factors determining the impact of care-giving on caregivers of elderly patients with dementia. A systematic literature review. *Maturitas, 66*(2), 191–200.

Schulz, R., & Beach, S. R. (1999). Caregiving as a risk factor for mortality: The caregiver health effects study. *Journal of the American Medical Association, 282*(23), 2215–2219.

Schulz, R., Boerner, K., Shear, K., Zhang, S., & Gitlin, L. S. (2006). Predictors of complicated grief among dementia caregivers: A prospective study of bereavement. *American Journal of Geriatric Psychiatry, 14*(8), 650–658.

Schulz, R., Mendelsohn, A. B., Haley, W., Mahoney, D., Allen, R. S., Zhang, S., Thompson, L., & Belle, S. (2003). End-of-life care and the effects of bereavement on family caregivers of persons with dementia. *New England Journal of Medicine, 349,* 1936–1942.

Svanberg, E., Spector, A., Stott, J. (2011). The impact of young onset dementia on the family: A literature review. *International Psychogeriatrics, 23*(3), 356–371.

Svanberg, E., Stott, J., & Spector, A. (2010). 'Just helping': Children living with a parent with young onset dementia. *Aging & Mental Health, 14*(6), 740–751.

van Vliet, D., de Vugt, M. E., Bakker, C., Koopmans, R. T., & Verhey, F. R. (2010). Impact of early onset dementia on caregivers: A review. *International Journal of Geriatric Psychiatry, 25*(11), 1091–1100.

Vitaliano, P. P., Murphy, M., Young, H. M., Echeverria, D., & Borson, S. (2011). Does caring for a spouse with dementia promote cognitive decline? A hypothesis and proposed mechanisms. *Journal of the American Geriatrics Society, 59*(5), 900–908.

Yeager, C. A., Hyer, L. A., Hobbs, B., & Coyne, A. C. (2010). Alzheimer's disease and vascular dementia: The complex relationship between diagnosis and caregiver burden. *Issues in Mental Health Nursing, 31*(6), 376–384.

Chapter 16

SUPPORTING CARERS

Jane Thompson
Australian National University

Chapter outcomes

When you have completed this chapter you will be able to:

▸ understand the many different approaches to supporting carers

▸ recognise the key components of the most effective interventions to support carers

▸ appreciate the complexity of needs among diverse carers.

Keywords

dementia carers, psychosocial interventions, support for carers

Introduction

As shown in Chapter 15, caring for a person with dementia exacts a significant toll on the carer's health and wellbeing. Much research has focused on specific interventions to prevent or alleviate these negative effects. Studies have been extensive, in part, because the declining ability of carers to cope is one of the strongest predictors of transition from home-based to institutional care. When the carer is coping better, not only is institutional placement delayed, but the care recipient may also do better.

Effectiveness of interventions may be influenced by many factors (Pinquart & Sorensen, 2006). Individualised interventions can be more easily adapted to the specific needs of carers and therefore may be more effective. However, group interventions are more effective in increasing social support. Because many dementia-related problems are difficult to change, longer interventions may be more effective. Carer age may also matter. Interventions that are effective for older carers may not necessarily work for younger carers. Further, because women generally provide more personal care and show higher levels of carer burden and depression than men, they may be more likely to benefit from interventions. Likewise, caregiving stressors may vary between spouses and adult children, with adult children more likely to experience role conflicts between caregiving and work. Thus, interventions may have different effects on spouse and adult child carers. Types of interventions can be classified as:

▶ interventions designed to support carers in their role
▶ interventions of formal approaches to care
▶ multi-component interventions.

Interventions designed to support carers in their role

Counselling and psychotherapy

Counselling can help carers resolve pre-existing personal problems that complicate caring, reduce conflicts between carers and the person being cared for and improve family relationships. Individual supportive counselling increases the time carers are able to provide care at home. Combining individual counselling with attending a support group is more beneficial in improving carers' mood and reducing depression than counselling alone (Dupuis, Epp & Smale, 2004; Goy, Kansagara & Freeman, 2010).

Individual and family counselling sessions tailored to each carer's specific situation and additional counselling on request improves carer depression symptoms. Family counselling can maximise the positive contributions of each member to caregiving; prevent one member from carrying the entire weight of the role; improve carers' understanding of how to ask for help; assist carers to determine what kind of help is reasonable to expect from family members; show carers how to accept help; and reduce family conflict (Joling et al., 2008).

The uptake of counselling services is often low and these services may not be accessed until later in the disease trajectory. Uptake can be increased when general practitioners actively recommend it to carers (Donath et al., 2010) and if counsellors actively contact carers to offer counselling (Grossfeld-Schmitz et al., 2010). Enhanced counselling during particular phases of the care journey, such as during the transition to residential care, is also helpful. While institutionalisation alone can reduce carer burden and depressive symptoms, carers who receive enhanced counselling can expect even greater reductions (Gaugler et al., 2008).

The effects of counselling vary with the skill level of the counsellor, the setting, the frequency and duration of contacts, and the training materials used. More intensive counselling using psychotherapeutic approaches either individually or group-based can help. For example, cognitive behaviourial therapy techniques help carers focus on identifying and modifying unproductive beliefs and behaviours and to develop new behaviours to deal with the demands and emotions of caring. Psychotherapy can improve carer burden, depression and anxiety (Sorensen et al., 2006). To enhance accessibility, psychotherapy can also be delivered using telecommunication technology (Czaja & Rubert, 2002).

One component of cognitive behaviourial therapy, cognitive reframing, may be particularly helpful (Vernooij-Dassen et al., 2011). This technique allows a person to take a situation and change the meaning they assign to it, thereby promoting adaptive behaviour. It targets certain beliefs about, for example, the carer's responsibilities to the person with dementia, their own need for support and why the person they care for behaves as they do. Cognitive reframing has the potential to reduce carers' anxiety, depression and stress.

Educational and skills training programs

Providing information can improve carers' quality of life as well as that of care recipients. Giving information alone (verbal or written) is not sufficient. Effective educational approaches include sessions with experts about the nature of the illness, its symptoms, causes and likely course; sessions identifying resources available for support; sessions focusing on effective management strategies for behaviour problems or agitation, communication skills and creating structure in daily routines; and sessions on stress management.

Dementia education programs give carers a sense of control and improve their ability to cope. When carers have attended educational sessions, transition to institutional care may be delayed and psychological wellbeing of the carer improved. Courses in stress management can lead to better awareness and understanding of stress and how to manage it, enhanced coping and reduced burden for carers. Education alone is probably not sufficient and a combination of education and support programs are more effective in reducing burden and enhancing carers' wellbeing (Dupuis, Epp & Smale, 2004).

More formal psycho-education (education about a certain situation or condition that causes psychological distress) involves the structured presentation of information about dementia care, generally in a group setting. It can include advice on ways of reducing stress, depression and anxiety and the provision of information on available resources, services and training for carers. It also creates a supportive environment to facilitate discussion of concerns and can include role-playing and other active learning techniques. Carers participating in such sessions have improved knowledge; reduced burden, depression, anger/hostility, fatigue and confusion; and show improvements in subjective wellbeing and in physical symptoms (Parker, Mills & Abbey, 2008). Psycho-educational interventions that include active participation of the carer and skill building (e.g. by combining educational components with homework and role-playing) are most effective. Such interventions may also improve the symptoms of the care recipient, perhaps by training the carer to redirect the person with dementia to avoid escalation of problem behaviour (Sorensen et al., 2006).

Targeting psycho-educational programs to meet expressed needs of carers is important. Training the carer to use behavioural management techniques with the person they care for reduces carer depressive symptoms and improves coping skills (Goy et al., 2010). Benefits may be greater if combined with additional components (e.g. self-care instructions for carers and/or exercise interventions for the care recipient). Strategies that focus on building resilience and positive coping skills, particularly in relation to managing challenging behaviours, are likely to bring the most gains for carers. Similarly, strategies to assist carers to communicate with the person with dementia and support memory and cognition are effective educational tools (Smith et al., 2011).

Educational programs for carers need to be targeted at issues appropriate to the stage of the caring journey. If the person with dementia moves into residential care, family–staff conflict can be a major stressor disturbing effective relationships and contributing to carer stress. Programs that involve information sharing and educational support for families, with the aim of developing constructive family–staff relationships, improve carer satisfaction and wellbeing, enhance the visiting experience for families and motivate the family to stay involved (Haesler, Bauer & Nay, 2010). Another novel educational program that may be beneficial at this stage involves the use of life stories to connect family and staff to people with dementia (Kellett et al., 2010).

Joint approaches involving both the carer and the person with dementia may also improve psychological outcomes for carers. For example, involving both parties in structured programs that teach the carer problem-solving skills has many benefits (Brodaty & Donkin, 2009). Another approach is reminiscence groups, run by professionals and volunteers, which use photographs, recordings and other objects to trigger personal memories (Woods et al., 2009). This improves relationships between people with dementia and their carers and benefits both.

Community-based occupational therapy programs for both carers and the person with dementia also improve care recipients' daily functioning and reduce the burden on the carer (Graff et al., 2006). Another joint approach works on reinforcing and strengthening the enriching aspects associated with the caring role. This is done through education programs aimed at adapting mutually enjoyable leisure activities to suit the person with dementia's capacity. Participation in such programs has positive benefits for carers including modifying their perception of their experience and bringing them to see their role as a positive opportunity rather than purely a burden (Carbonneau, Caron & Desrosiers, 2011).

Support groups and other forms of social support

Where providing emotional support for carers is the main focus of interventions, this has typically been provided through support groups based on a mutual support model. These groups focus on building rapport among members. They provide the opportunity to share personal feelings and concerns and to discuss caregiving experiences, common problems and solutions. Participation helps to overcome feelings of social isolation often experienced by carers (Chien et al., 2011; Grassel et al., 2010).

Support groups may be professionally led or peer-led and unstructured. Experts may be invited occasionally to provide medical, legal or other information. Telecommunication and computer-based technology may also be used as a means of connecting groups of carers for mutual support.

Carers who have been members of ongoing support groups indicate that their capacity to manage and cope with their day-to-day concerns is strongly influenced by their support group experience (Brown & Tweedie, 2005, 2007). Members who attend sessions on a regular basis experience the most positive outcomes. The experience of grief and loss is a profound commonality shared by group members and the way this is managed by the individual and the group is influenced strongly by the skills and experience of the group leader. The desire to access education and information about dementia and service options may be the main impetus for support group membership. However, long-term members state that the mutual aid they give to, and receive from, other members is paramount and often becomes the main reason for continued membership.

Support groups can be run successfully by telephone, which may be particularly useful for carers who are housebound, geographically isolated or do not want to participate in face-to-face groups (Shanley et al., 2004). They may also benefit carers from culturally diverse backgrounds.

There are other effective forms of social support for carers including befriending schemes where volunteers provide emotional support for matched carers through companionship and conversation (Charlesworth et al., 2008). Carers enjoy and gain from the experience, particularly if befriended by former carers. Another is the 'Alzheimer's Cafe' where the person with dementia and their carer, family member or friend attend.

The service promotes social inclusion, prevents isolation and improves the social and emotional wellbeing of attendees (Dow et al., 2011).

The benefits of social support for carers are not to be underestimated. The more social support carers receive prior to the death of the person with dementia, the better adjusted they may be post-bereavement.

Respite from caring

Respite is designed to give temporary rest, time out or relief to carers through the provision of substitute care for the person with dementia (Lee & Cameron, 2004). Respite allows the carer to take leave from their caregiving responsibilities, to distance themselves from their caregiving identity and connect with a different world. Carers need to engage with their alternative selves to have true breaks from caring (de la Cuesta-Benjumea, 2010, 2011).

Respite can be delivered in the home, as a centre-based day program or in a residential institutional setting. It may involve overnight or daytime-only care with care providers who are trained, untrained or volunteers. The care may be for couple of hours to a number of weeks. It may be on a regular basis involving a certain number of weekly hours or days, planned or unplanned. Vacation or emergency respite provides round-the-clock substitute care for a short-term stay when the carer goes on holiday, is temporarily ill or when other personal or family demands interfere with, or preclude, the care of the person with dementia. Carers may also access informal types of respite care such as help from family and friends. Alternative types of respite suit different carer and family needs at different times with varying advantages and drawbacks.

Providing respite for carers is generally aimed at preventing or postponing permanent placement of the person with dementia in long-term residential care through shoring up their carers' physical and mental health. The reduction in stress to the carer, produced by a temporary relief from care-giving, should also allow the person with dementia to have a better relationship with their carer and to receive better care while in the community.

While respite care services are important to give carers a break they must also create social activity and engagement for the person with dementia. The periods of respite can also be used to offer professional re-evaluation of the needs of the person with dementia and to provide rehabilitation.

There is limited evidence for the benefits of respite in terms of carer wellbeing (Goy et al., 2010; Pinquart & Sorensen, 2006); however, carers value respite services very highly with increased availability and flexibility of respite care being common requests in surveys. Carers do need assurance that quality care is being given to the person with dementia before they can experience the temporary relief from worry and stress that the respite intends to provide.

Exercise programs

One reason carers experience negative health outcomes may be because they are less likely to engage in preventative health behaviours such as regular physical activity. Older carers and those experiencing high levels of burden find it particularly difficult to participate in leisure-time physical activities and to access community-based programs (Hirano et al., 2011b). Home-based, physical activity regimens are an alternative and provide a promising strategy for increasing physical activity among carers (Hirano et al., 2011a). Programs including a nutritional component may also have added benefit (Castro et al., 2002).

Individually tailored exercise interventions that target both the person with dementia and their carer may suit carers who prefer to do things with the person they care for rather than having services directed at either one or the other (Cerga-Pashoja et al., 2010).

Assistive technologies

Assistive technologies include electronic or computerised devices or systems designed to help carers monitor and supervise persons with dementia. They can help the person with dementia to function more easily, independently and safely and reduce carer stress and burden. They may also enable the person with dementia to live longer in their own home.

There is a wide range of commercially available and emerging assistive technologies that have potential applications for people with dementia and their carers, but a limited amount of rigorous research involving their use has been done and there are some ethical concerns (Zwijsen, Niemeijer & Hertogh, 2011). However, improvements in different aspects of carer wellbeing have been found in some studies (Bharucha et al., 2009; Goy et al., 2010). There are many examples of assistive technologies that might be useful and may help to make carers' lives easier and free up time for self. Examples include installations in the home that use web-based monitoring systems with cameras and power, as well as water and door sensors. Global positioning systems (GPS) are also effective, reliable and successful in detecting wandering, locating lost persons with dementia and reducing carer stress and possibly burden and depression. Another example is the use of electronic calendars, which enable persons with dementia to be more oriented to the date and time of day and can also reduce repeated questions to the carer, thereby improving wellbeing for both (O'Keeffe, Maier & Freiman, 2010). One last example is night monitoring systems, which can assist carers in preventing night time injuries and unattended home exits in care recipients and may result in improved sleep patterns of carers (Rowe et al., 2009).

Interventions of formal approaches to care

Advance care planning

Throughout the dementia care journey, many decisions about the care of the person with dementia involve proxy decision-making by carers. Difficult decisions often have to be made at times of crisis and great stress. The burden of responsibility placed on carers to act as proxy decision-makers is enormous. In particular, towards the end of the life of the person with dementia most carers find themselves in the unenviable situation of both grieving for the anticipated loss of that person and being required to make difficult decisions on their behalf. The ethical burden on carers 'to do the right thing' may contribute to the already distressed carer and they need support from experienced and educated health professionals (Ashton et al., 2011).

The importance of having Advance Care Plans reflecting the wishes of the person with dementia has been discussed in Chapter 14. While these aid decision-making, there may be times when plans conflict with the carers' own wishes and priorities. Regarding end-of-life decisions in residential care facilities, carers are faced with the need for particularly complex proxy decision-making. This difficult process can be assisted by frequent contact with staff, who can offer empathy, reassurance, understanding, guidance and communication. Carers often feel uncomfortable in their decision-making role and can express feelings of stress, guilt, fear, doubt and anxiety. In addition, carers are a diverse group and not all will wish to have the same level of engagement in decision-making (Sanders et al., 2009).

Palliative approach to dementia care

Death is a difficult subject for most carers and families to discuss or plan for, but a poor quality of life for their loved one during the progression of the disease and in the process of dying is distressing (Hines et al., 2011). A palliative approach to care at the end of life, as discussed in detail in Chapter 14, is both appropriate and effective in terms of benefit to patients and their carers. When a person is dying with advanced dementia the needs of families and carers are unique. They require significant extra support during the advanced stages of the disease and place high value on psychosocial support and holistic care at this time.

Models of care

Dementia is a complex disease requiring a multidisciplinary model of care to deal with its complex range of mental, physical and social problems.

Case management models have positive effects including a decrease in behavioural and psychological symptoms in the person with dementia; a reduction in carer distress, burden and depression; deferred placement of the person with dementia into residential care; and an increased use of community services by both carers and the person being cared for (Goy et al., 2010; Low, Yap & Brodaty, 2011).

Case management by specialist dementia care nurses is a model widely promoted in the UK. Nurses work primarily with the carers, focus exclusively on dementia and offer continuing involvement with emotional support, provision of information and coordination of practical support. Carers receiving the service show greater improvements in levels of anxiety and insomnia than those receiving conventional services (Woods et al., 2003).

Consumer-directed care enables care recipients and their carers, to the extent they are capable and wish to do so, to make choices about the types of services they access and the delivery of those services, including who will deliver them and when. It can improve satisfaction with care and community service use, with no adverse effect on clinical outcomes (Low et al., 2011; Tilly & Rees, 2007).

In-home models of care with support from community-based services are common. A carer's decision to provide care at home, with assistance of formal services, depends on many factors, not least of which are availability and cost. Providing in-home care, particularly until the end of the life of the person with dementia, is a challenging task necessitating extensive formal support services. Challenges include forming and maintaining relationships with paid carers and obtaining adequate, appropriate, consistent, sufficient and flexible services (Ward-Griffin et al., 2012).

More research is needed on best models of care to address the special needs of specific cultural groups; carers in same-sex-relationships; indigenous populations; younger onset dementia carers; and carers of people with both dementia and an intellectual disability. Individually tailored, culturally sensitive programs are likely to be effective.

Design of residential facilities

The design of the physical environment is an important contributor to the quality of dementia care. Small, home-like environments are beneficial for both people with dementia and their carers (Smit et al., 2011; Verbeek et al., 2010). Such facilities, while safe and familiar, are also likely to provide a social and/or professional environment conducive to quality care. When persons with dementia reside in small-scale environments, carers have reported less burden and higher satisfaction with nursing staff compared with those whose care recipients reside in regular nursing homes. Psychological distress among carers may show greater decline during the first six months after admission if the person they care for is admitted to a small-scale facility.

Multi-component interventions

Multi-component interventions combine components from different interventions such as education, support and respite. They are also tailored to individual needs of the carer-care recipient dyad and tend to have a greater effect than a single intervention focusing on a particular issue.

A model program is the US Resources for Enhancing Alzheimer's Caregiver Health (REACH): an individualised multi-component home and telephone-based intervention aimed at enhancing carers' coping skills and management of dementia-related behaviours (Goy et al., 2010; Nichols et al., 2008). The program has been evaluated in diverse populations and involves trained staff making home visits, telephone calls and offering structured telephone support sessions. The strategies include information sharing, instruction, role-playing, problem-solving, skills training, stress management techniques and telephone support groups. Participation significantly improves carers' quality of life in terms of burden; depression and emotional wellbeing; self-care and healthy behaviours; social support; and management of care recipient problem behaviours. It also decreases the amount of time carers are required to provide direct care, giving them much needed respite. Institutional placement of care recipients, therefore, may be slightly delayed. Taking part in the program helps carers feel more confident in working with the person with dementia, makes life easier for them, improves their ability to provide care and improves the care recipient's life.

Practical advice and tips

Getting organised and connected
Once a diagnosis of dementia has been made most carers will find themselves on a very unfamiliar pathway. They will need to access all the help they possibly can.

A good start to getting organised for the journey ahead is to contact the local Alzheimer's Association who can provide information, emotional support and counselling and practical advice; offer support groups and training programs; and enable carers to find out what their entitlements are and about local services. Carers associations also support carers, deliver carer programs and services and advocate on behalf of all carers.

Accessing appropriate care

Carers benefit most from an integrated, multidisciplinary model of care that either is coordinated by a case manager (who may be a dementia specialist) or may be consumer directed. Such models may not be available to all carers; however, if possible it would be advisable to try and access such an arrangement.

If they are to provide care at home, carers will need assistance so they should seek services that are available, appropriate, consistent, flexible and sufficient. Many carers do not have sufficient resources themselves (or access to them), the time or the skills to continue home-based care until the end stage when the person with dementia has high-care needs. Whether carers can manage at home will depend very much on compliance of the person cared for and on other demands on the carer.

If choosing residential care, carers need to be assured that positive family–staff relationships will be fostered and there will be support for ongoing involvement of carers. Choosing a well-designed facility is important, although they may not always be available.

Making plans for the future

It is very difficult early on to comprehend that this journey will involve the loss of capacity and subsequent death of the person with dementia. Carers at the end of the journey often say that they wished they had understood this or that someone had made it clearer. Setting up the legal arrangements for the carer to become a proxy decision-maker in all matters for the person with dementia, including medical decision-making, is critical and needs to be done early.

It is also important to think about making formal plans in relation to end-of-life health care for the person with dementia. Ascertaining their wishes early on in the illness is important and an appropriate form of instruction can be prepared for medical staff and designated family members about end-of-life management. Advance care planning is a distressing activity needing the support of experienced and educated health professionals.

Carers also need to make some plans for their own future. Planning will depend very much on the stage of life of the carer, especially in regards to maintaining a presence in the paid workforce. My own counsellor strongly encouraged me to keep up part-time work if I possibly could. This proved very valuable, as I was able to continue with work I enjoyed, which gave me an identity beyond being a carer. After my husband died I then had a role I could continue.

Shoring up social and emotional supports

Social and emotional support is essential if carers are to survive the dementia caring journey. Accessing multiple sources of support is likely to be beneficial if carers are to avoid social isolation and the potential loneliness of the long distance carer.

Regular attendance at a small, ongoing support group with a skilled and experienced group leader is likely to help. Finding the right support group, or groups, with carers who are able to develop good rapport with each other is important. My local Alzheimer's Association recognised the need for a support group specifically for younger women (under 65) caring for a partner with dementia. This was, and still is, an enormous source of support.

Computer and telephone-mediated support groups may also be effective particularly for carers isolated by distance or who are housebound. Local carer or Alzheimer's groups may be able to link individual carers with each other. Attending a social group that engages both the carer and the person with dementia, such as an Alzheimer's Cafe (if available), may also help.

Seeking emotional support early in the journey, through individual counselling with a counsellor skilled in psychotherapeutic techniques, may help, as may family counselling if necessary. Combining individual counselling with attending a support group may be more beneficial than counselling alone. Counselling sessions tailored to each carer's situation and enhanced counselling during particular phases of the journey – for example, the transition to residential care, during the dying phase and after death – may also help.

Getting information and skills training

Carers need to know as much as they possibly can about the new world they are entering as a carer. Numerous printed and electronic resources are available. Books based on personal experiences are likely to assist (e.g. Tom Valenta's book *Remember Me, Mrs V?: Caring for my Wife: Her Alzheimer's and Others' Stories* and Sue Pieters-Hawke's *Hazel's Journey: A Personal Experience of Alzheimer's*).

Attending group educational or skills training programs is likely to help, especially if targeted to particular needs in the various stages of the journey. Programs combining both education and support with active participation of the carer are best. Individualised skills training may be appropriate for some carers with specific needs. Joint approaches involving both the person with dementia and the carer if appropriate may also assist.

Taking respite from caring

Carers value respite very highly, with many saying they could not cope without it. There are many ways of providing respite and it is important to find what works best for the carer and the person with dementia.

Be reassured that it is legitimate for carers to have a rest but carers need to be satisfied with the quality of care given by the substitute care provider. It is also important to find services that are flexible, accessible and targeted to specific needs, which will vary at different stages of the journey.

Using assistive technologies

Carers may need to introduce products that incorporate assistive technologies on a trial basis and determine for themselves whether they are both effective and beneficial. Examples include monitoring devices and sensors installed in the home, location systems (GPS) worn by the person with dementia and electronic calendars to assist with orientation to time of day.

Looking after carers' health and wellbeing

It is absolutely critical for carers to look after their own health and wellbeing, but it is perhaps the hardest step of all. Carers will need help in meeting the fundamental needs for sleep, a healthy diet and exercise. Exercise, with or without the care recipient, either in a community-based setting or even delivered at home, has benefits for carers. Getting enough sleep is also important, but can be difficult, particularly if carers are disturbed at night by the person with dementia. Accessing overnight care services may be necessary to provide restorative sleep. Seeking help with management of night time disturbances may also help.

Liz, who was a carer for her husband John, describes well what helped her to look after herself:

> I was a carer for my husband with younger onset dementia. The most helpful thing for me was to have one day off a week where I went walking with a walking group. This enabled me to get exercise, fresh air and stimulating conversation with other walkers. John lost the ability to communicate early on so initially I found it great to be able to join in proper conversations. As his illness progressed and it became more demanding, I was too tired to debate or argue about everyday things but it was still great to listen in and hear others talk about TV programs, newspaper articles, family news and so on. It becomes very isolating when you are a full-time carer so this was a special time when I could recharge. My caseworker ensured that I always had the time off to walk, which was great.

Conclusion

Unpaid dementia carers need help and support to carry out their caring role; however, many do not have access to services or are reluctant to ask for help and use available services. Current best practice is for them to be offered an assessment of their emotional, psychological and social needs and, if accepted, receive multi-component tailored interventions to address those needs, which will change throughout the journey. Interventions may include:

- individual or group psycho-education
- peer-support groups tailored to the needs of the individual
- telephone and internet information and support
- training courses about dementia, services and benefits and dementia-care problem-solving
- psychological therapy (including cognitive behavioural therapy) with a specialist practitioner if required
- access to appropriate respite.

The provision of preventative supports, rather than resorting to costly patient care for carers who reach the point of burnout and for care recipients who have been institutionalised, makes enormous common, let alone economic, sense.

References

Ashton, S., Roe, B., Jack, B., & McClelland, B. (2011). A study to explore the experience of advanced care planning among family caregivers and relatives of people with advanced dementia. *BMJ Supportive & Palliative Care, 1,* 65–109.

Bharucha, A. J., Anand, V., Forlizzi, J., Dew, M. A., Reynolds, C. F., Stevens, S., & Wactlar, H. (2009). Intelligent assistive technology applications to dementia care: current capabilities, limitations, and future challenges. *American Journal of Geriatric Psychiatry, 17*(2), 88–104.

Brodaty, H., & Donkin, M. (2009). Family caregivers of people with dementia. *Dialogues in Clinical Neuroscience, 11*(2), 217–228.

Brown, J., & Tweedie, R. (2005). *Quality support groups research project: A report on dementia support groups in New South Wales. Phase I: A literature review, leaders' perspectives and group composition.* North Ryde, NSW: Alzheimer's Australia NSW.

Brown, J., & Tweedie, R. (2007). *Quality support groups research project: a report on dementia support groups in New South Wales. Phase II: A literature review, leaders' perspectives and group composition.* North Ryde, NSW: Alzheimer's Australia NSW.

Carbonneau, H., Caron, C. D., & Desrosiers J. (2011). Effects of an adapted leisure education program as a means of support for caregivers of people with dementia. *Archives of Gerontology and Geriatrics, 53*(1), 31–39.

Castro, C. M., Wilcox, S., O'Sullivan, P., Baumann K., & King A. C. (2002). An exercise program for women who are caring for relatives with dementia. *Psychosomatic Medicine, 64*(3), 458–468.

Cerga-Pashoja, A., Lowery, D., Bhattacharya, R., Griffin, M., Iliffe, S., Lee, J., Leonard, C., Ricketts, S., Strother, L., Waters, F., Ritchie, C. W., & Warner, J. (2010). Evaluation of exercise on individuals with dementia and their carers: a randomised controlled trial. *Trials, 11*, 53.

Charlesworth, G., Shepstone, L., Wilson E., Thalanany, M., Mugford, M., & Poland, F. (2008). Does befriending by trained lay workers improve psychological well-being and quality of life for carers of people with dementia, and at what cost? A randomised controlled trial. *Health Technology Assessment, 12*(4), 1–78.

Chien, L. Y., Chu, H., Guo, J. L., Liao, Y. M., Chang, L. I., Chen, C. H., & Chou, K. R. (2011). Caregiver support groups in patients with dementia: a meta-analysis. *International Journal of Geriatric Psychiatry, 26*(10), 1089–1098.

Czaja, S. J., & Rubert, M. P. (2002). Telecommunications technology as an aid to family caregivers of persons with dementia. *Psychosomatic Medicine, 64*(3), 469–476.

de la Cuesta-Benjumea, C. (2010). The legitimacy of rest: conditions for the relief of burden in advanced dementia care-giving. *Journal of Advanced Nursing, 66*(5), 988–998.

de la Cuesta-Benjumea, C. (2011). Strategies for the relief of burden in advanced dementia care-giving. *Journal of Advanced Nursing, 67*, 1790–1799.

Donath, C., Grassel, E., Grossfeld-Schmitz, M., Menn, P., Lauterberg, J., Wunder, S., Marx, P., Ruckdäschel, S., Mehlig, H., & Holle, R. (2010). Effects of general practitioner training and family support services on the care of home-dwelling dementia patients – results of a controlled cluster-randomized study. *BMC Health Services Research, 10*, 314.

Dow, B., Haralambous, B., Hempton, C., Hunt, S., & Calleja, D. (2011). Evaluation of Alzheimer's Australia Vic Memory Lane Cafes. *International Psychogeriatrics, 23*(2), 246–255.

Dupuis, S. L., Epp, T., & Smale, B. (2004). *Caregivers of persons with dementia: Roles, experiences, supports, and coping. A literature review.* Waterloo, Canada: Murray Alzheimer Research and Education Program, University of Waterloo.

Gaugler, J. E., Roth, D. L., Haley W. E., & Mittelman, M. S. (2008). Can counseling and support reduce burden and depressive symptoms in caregivers of people with Alzheimer's disease during the transition to institutionalization? Results from the New York University caregiver intervention study. *Journal of the American Geriatric Society, 56*(3), 421–428.

Goy, E., Kansagara, D., & Freeman, M. (2010). *A Systematic Evidence Review of Interventions for Nonprofessional Caregivers of Individuals with Dementia,* VA-ESP Project #05-225. Washington, DC: Department of Veteran Affairs.

Graff, M. J., Vernooij-Dassen, M. J., Thijssen, M., Dekker, J., Hoefnagels, W. H., & Olde Rikkert, M. G. (2006). Community based occupational therapy for patients with dementia and their care givers: Randomised controlled trial. *BMJ, 333*(7580), 1196–1199. doi:10.1136/bmj.39001.688843.BE

Grassel, E., Trilling, A., Donath, C., & Luttenberger, K. (2010). Support groups for dementia caregivers – predictors for utilisation and expected quality from a family caregiver's point of view: A questionnaire survey Part I. *BMC Health Services Research, 10*, 219.

Grossfeld-Schmitz, M., Donath, C., Holle, R., Lauterberg, J., Ruckdaeschel, S., Mehlig, H., Marx, P., Wunder, S., & Gräßel, E. (2010). Counsellors contact dementia caregivers – predictors of utilisation in a longitudinal study. *BMC Geriatrics, 10*(1), 24.

Haesler, E., Bauer, M., & Nay, R. (2010). Recent evidence on the development and maintenance of constructive staff-family relationships in the care of older people – a report on a systematic review update. *International Journal of Evidence-Based Healthcare, 8*(2), 45–74.

Hines, S., McCrow, J., Abbey, J., Foottit, J., Wilson, J., Franklin, S., Beattie, E. (2011). The effectiveness and appropriateness of a palliative approach to care for people with advanced dementia: a systematic review. *JBI Database of Systematic Reviews, 9*(26), 960–1131.

Hirano, A., Suzuki, Y., Kuzuya, M., Onishi, J., Ban, N., & Umegaki, H. (2011a). Influence of regular exercise on subjective sense of burden and physical symptoms in community-dwelling caregivers of dementia patients: a randomized controlled trial. *Archives of Gerontology & Geriatrics, 53*(2), e158–e163.

Hirano, A., Suzuki, Y., Kuzuya, M., Onishi, J., Hasegawa, J., Ban, N., & Umegaki, H. (2011b). Association between the caregiver's burden and physical activity in community-dwelling caregivers of dementia patients. *Archives of Gerontology & Geriatrics, 52*(3), 295–298.

Joling, K. J., van Hout, H. P., Scheltens, P., Vernooij-Dassen, M., van den Berg, B., Bosmans, J., Gillissen, F., Mittelman, M., & van Marwijk, H. W. (2008). (Cost)-effectiveness of family meetings on indicated prevention of anxiety and depressive symptoms and disorders of primary family caregivers of patients with dementia: design of a randomized controlled trial. *BMC Geriatrics, 8*, 2.

Kellett, U., Moyle, W., McAllister, M., King, C., & Gallagher, F. (2010). Life stories and biography: A means of connecting family and staff to people with dementia. *Journal of Clinical Nursing, 19*(11–12), 1707–1715.

Lee, H., & Cameron, M. (2004). Respite care for people with dementia and their carers. *Cochrane Database of Systematic Reviews, 2004*(1), Art. No.: CD004396.

Low, L. F., Yap, M., & Brodaty, H. (2011). A systematic review of different models of home and community care services for older persons. *BMC Health Services Research, 11*, 93.

Nichols, L. O., Chang, C., Lummus, A., Burns, R., Martindale-Adams, J., Graney, M. J., Coon, D. W., & Czaja, S. (2008). The cost-effectiveness of a behavior intervention with caregivers of patients with Alzheimer's disease. *Journal of the American Geriatric Society, 56*(3), 413–420.

O'Keeffe, J., Maier, J., & Freiman, M. (2010). *Assistive technology for people with dementia and their caregivers at home: What might help.* Washington, DC: Administration on Aging.

Parker, D., Mills, S., & Abbey, J. (2008). Effectiveness of interventions that assist caregivers to support people with dementia living in the community: A systematic review. *International Journal of Evidence Based Healthcare, 6*(2), 137–172.

Pinquart, M., & Sorensen, S. (2006). Helping caregivers of persons with dementia: which interventions work and how large are their effects? *International Psychogeriatrics, 18*(4), 577–595.

Rowe, M. A., Kelly, A., Horne, C., Lane, S., Campbell, J., Lehman, B., Phipps, C., Keller, M., Pe Benito, A. (2009). Reducing dangerous nighttime events in persons with dementia by using a nighttime monitoring system. *Alzheimer's Dementia, 5*(5), 419–426.

Sanders, S., Butcher, H. K., Swails, P., & Power, J. (2009). Portraits of caregivers of end-stage dementia patients receiving hospice care. *Death Studies, 33*(6), 521–556.

Shanley, C., Roddy, M., Cruysmans, B., & Eisenberg, M. (2004). The humble telephone: A medium for running carer support groups. *Australasian Journal on Ageing, 23*(2), 82–85.

Smit, D., te Boekhorst, S., de Lange, J., Depla, M. F., Eefsting, J. A., & Pot, A. M. (2011). The long-term effect of group living homes versus regular nursing homes for people with dementia on psychological distress of informal caregivers. *Aging & Mental Health, 15*(5), 557–561.

Smith, E. R., Broughton, M., Baker, R., Pachana, N. A., Angwin, A. J., Humphreys, M. S., Mitchell, L., Byrne, G. J., Copland, D. A., Gallois, C., Hegney, D., & Chenery, H. J. (2011). Memory and communication support in dementia: Research-based strategies for caregivers. *International Psychogeriatrics, 23*(2), 256–263.

Sorensen, S., Duberstein, P., Gill, D., & Pinquart, M. (2006). Dementia care: Mental health effects, intervention strategies, and clinical implications. *Lancet Neurology, 5*(11), 961–973.

Tilly, J., & Rees, G. (2007). *Consumer-directed care. A way to empower consumers?* Alzheimer's Australia Paper 11. Canberra: Alzheimer's Australia.

Verbeek, H., Zwakhalen, S. M., van Rossum, E., Ambergen, T., Kempen, G. I., & Hamers, J. P. (2010). Small-scale, homelike facilities versus regular psychogeriatric nursing home wards: A cross-sectional study into residents' characteristics. *BMC Health Services Research, 10*, 30.

Vernooij-Dassen, M., Draskovic, I., McCleery, J., & Downs, M. (2011). Cognitive reframing for carers of people with dementia. *Cochrane Database of Systematic Reviews, 9*(11), CD005318.

Ward-Griffin, C., Hall, J., DeForge, R., St-Amant, O., McWilliam, C., Oudshoorn, A., Forbes, D., & Klosek, M. (2012). Dementia home care resources: How are we managing? *Journal of Aging Research, 2012*(2012): 590724.

Woods, R., Wills, W., Higginson, I. J., Hobbins, J., & Whitby, M.(2003). Support in the community for people with dementia and their carers: a comparative outcome study of specialist mental-health service interventions. *International Journal of Geriatric Psychiatry, 18*(4), 298–307.

Woods, R. T., Bruce, E., Edwards, R., Hounsome, B., Keady, J., Moniz-Cook, E. D., Orrell, M., & Russell, I. T. (2009). Reminiscence groups for people with dementia and their family carers: pragmatic eight-centre randomised trial of joint reminiscence and maintenance versus usual treatment: A protocol. *Trials, 10,* 64.

Zwijsen, S. A., Niemeijer, A. R., & Hertogh, C. M. (2011). Ethics of using assistive technology in the care for community-dwelling elderly people: An overview of the literature. *Aging & Mental Health, 15*(4), 419–427.